THE GIFT

THE
GIFT

Learning to Appreciate the Value of Life

Dwayne Bray

LONGSTREET
Atlanta, Georgia

Published by
LONGSTREET PRESS
2140 Newmarket Parkway
Suite 122
Marietta, GA 30067
www.longstreetpress.net

Some portions of this text have been adapted from articles that first appeared in the *Dayton Daily News*, in particular a series of stories written by Laura Dempsey.

Printed in the United States of America

2nd printing 2000

Library of Congress Catalog Card Number: 99-60102

ISBN: 1-56352-535-6

Jacket and surgery photographs by Jim Witmer, the *Dayton Daily News*.

Jacket design by Burtch Hunter
Book design by Megan Wilson

DEDICATION

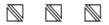

For Natalie, Dwayne Jr.,
Christian, and Albert.

ACKNOWLEDGMENTS

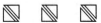

For this book, I thank God.

I also thank two of my very special teachers at Shaw High School, Dean Ulsenheimer and Lori Urogdy. I have had many journalism mentors and editors, and none have been more caring than Donna Rouner, Leo Jeffres, Steve Sidlo, and Bill Overend. My editors at Longstreet Press, Chuck Perry and Tysie Whitman, have shown great patience and exceptional insights throughout this project. A number of folks at the *Dayton Daily News* encouraged this book and provided a kind word and gentle prodding: Thanks Ron Rollins, J. Frazier Smith, Nichelle Smith, Mary McCarty, Sean McClelland, Laura Dempsey, and Jim Witmer.

I'm also grateful for the encouragement I receive from my grandmother, whose faith never wavers. And from my mother, who has shown me that one can reclaim her life from evil forces and become a true role model. Finally, I want to thank Calvin, his wife, Misha, and their children for their support. Calvin, may you live to be old and gray.

THE GIFT

PROLOGUE

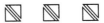

Calvin is going to die. I just know it. Don't tell me that his dialysis treatments, three times a week, will keep him alive. Some people with kidney disease make it years on dialysis, but Calvin won't. I just feel it. Too many times his blood has clotted during the treatments. Too many times he has gone to University Hospitals of Cleveland with the intention of taking life-sustaining dialysis, only to be rushed into surgery to have a new shunt placed in his arm or leg. That's no way to live.

That's why I am here at University myself, in a hospital gown. Over the past year the nurses have poked and prodded me. They have taken so much blood for testing that I'm surprised I have any left. They have given me an ultrasound. They have run a catheter through an incision in my thigh. They have shot dye into my kidneys, taken X-rays of them, and deemed me fit.

Fit to be here on July 8, 1997. I am giving Calvin one of my kidneys. I am giving him life. Many times in our pasts, we risked our lives for nothing more than perceived pride or even a cheap thrill. But now it seems so very valuable, so worth the risk we're taking.

I lie here on this hospital bed surrounded by nurses and doctors and technicians and other patients who are preparing for surgeries of their own. I lie here surrounded by friends and family, some who understand my decision to donate to my cousin, some who don't.

Standing by my bed is Natalie, my wife. Her support is needed, even though she really doesn't want me to go through with this operation. The two women standing between the beds are grandmothers—the one with the shawl draped over her shoulders is Sangenella Smith, Calvin's and my maternal grandmother, and the one talking to her is Calvin's paternal grandmother, Emma Pearl Davis.

The petite woman who just breezed out of this pre-op room is Dorothy Brimage, our mothers' sister. My mother can't be here because she is in Houston, a recovering heroin addict trying to get back on her feet. Her sister, Calvin's mother, is about two miles from this hospital in the Cuyahoga County Jail, locked up after another theft offense spurred by her own two-decade-long heroin habit.

Calvin and I grew up in an extended family, and you always learn that even if the people who are supposed to be with you during a crisis aren't there, someone else will take their place. That's what large families are about. In this case, Debra Dennis is here with us as well. She is Calvin's godmother. She is the one with the dark turban wrapped around her head, standing close to Calvin's bed. That young lady with her, the one in her early twenties, is Shamone, her daughter, just another pillar of support. Oh, I almost forgot the young woman holding Calvin's hand. That's his wife, Misha. She is also the mother of his two children, one born just six months ago.

There are no male relatives among our well-wishers,

for we are from a matriarchal family. Women are the ones who stick by you in a time of need.

The anesthesia is starting to take effect. I tell the doctors that I'm ready to go. Trying to be as brave as others insist I am, I say, Let's do it.

The year-long wait for this surgery is over. I am now inside the operating room. Drs. Rajiv Tewari and Sheila Vaz place a mask over my mouth. They are the anesthesiologists, feeding their drug to me. Seconds later, I am unconscious, paralyzed, at their mercy.

But I have faith I will be all right, and so will Calvin. He will be a new man.

If all goes well.

PART

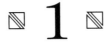

1

The youngest grandmother in the world, that's what some people are calling her. She is only thirty-one, and it is 1964, a time when most other new grandmothers are in their early forties, at the least. Sangenella doesn't want to be a grandmother, that's for sure. Queenie, her thirteen-year-old daughter, had seen this older boy hanging out on the corner by Hough Junior High School. One day he kissed her. She started skipping classes, going over to his house to drink Thunderbird. They told each other they were in love. That's why Sangenella is a grandmother.

She didn't like it, but by the time Queenie gives birth, Sangenella knows it's time to move forward. The sight of a newborn has a way of taking the edge off a difficult situation. Sangenella knows when a baby comes into the family, it is time for everyone to work together and help raise the child. Not fight over his presence. Not argue about who should not have gotten pregnant. That won't do any good. The arrival of a new kid means it is time to move on, and that is what she plans to do. It's why she is riding the No. 3 Superior bus to downtown Cleveland.

The bus will take her to a meeting with her welfare case-worker. She hopes to get her monthly check raised so she can support the baby.

◩

The No. 3 is quiet and all that can be heard is the rev of the engine and the squeak of the brakes. The trip will take about twenty-five minutes, and Sangenella glances out the window at the ethnic Cleveland neighborhoods in her path. She is in awe of the elaborate churches with looming Gothic spires. She admires the buildings' architecture for their towering strength and their ability to last, never looking worn, always standing tall. She just wishes she could find a man with those same qualities and not the kind who wants to leave her at the first sign of trouble. She laughs at the thought, knowing full well that her daydreaming is only a way to keep her mind off the dreaded meeting with the caseworker.

The bus halts to a stop at downtown Public Square—rather abruptly, jarring her back to reality. Sangenella gets off the bus and sees the historic Soldiers and Sailors Monument across the windswept square. She marvels at the elegance of the Terminal Tower, once the world's tallest building.

A somewhat stout, if not beautiful, brown-skinned woman, she fastens her old, frayed coat and starts the two-block walk to the red-brick welfare building on St. Clair Avenue. This building has a way of scaring poor, undereducated women like Sangenella, whose mistakes, or those of their children, bring them here, seeking public assistance.

THE GIFT

Sangenella has a seat in the waiting room after taking a number. Soon she hears a stern voice: Sangenella Brimage! Brimage is the name of her second husband, from whom she is separated and plans to divorce. The bark in the caseworker's voice is indicative of her lack of patience with Sangenella's predicament, a need for extra benefits and food stamps. The caseworker advises her that adoption is the best route for a baby with such a young mother and an overwhelmed grandmother who already is raising seven children of her own. Neither Queenie nor Sangenella has a spouse to help offset these expenses. Sangenella has a live-in boyfriend. But she wouldn't tell the caseworker about him—women on welfare know cohabitation is a sure way to get their checks cut off.

The caseworker's patience grows shorter. She tells Sangenella that plenty of families are looking to adopt healthy newborns, even black ones. The baby would have a good life with a strong, two-parent family, and maybe even some brothers and sisters. He would have a nice home, not Sangenella's cluttered, rodent-infested apartment. He would have all the amenities in life that Sangenella can't afford.

The caseworker says, You can't take care of yourself and the seven children you already have, Mrs. Brimage.

Sangenella shifts in her chair, clinging to her oversized purse as if it contains one million dollars and the end to all her worries. Squeezing it gives her comfort in this otherwise uneasy, one-sided confrontation. How are you going to take care of another child, Mrs. Brimage? the casework barks once more.

Sangenella shivers. I ain't giving up my own blood, she

responds meekly. The Lord, that's how. The Lord gonna take care of us.

When she leaves the welfare building she is spent. But she was able to acquire a slight raise that brings her monthly check now to more than three hundred dollars.

◩

Sangenella is my mother's mother. I was born on October 18, 1964. For years after my birth, we live in various apartments overrun by large cockroaches and rats. Our fortunes change dramatically in January 1967, when one of Grandma's elder sisters knocks on the door of our overcrowded apartment on Lakeview Avenue on Cleveland's East Side.

Aunt Laura has always been the most business savvy of Grandma's eight sisters and brothers. That was evident after their mother died and Aunt Laura had to take care of her four younger sisters and brothers who were still living on the family farm in Cecil, Alabama. When Aunt Laura was old enough, she left the farm and returned several years later to take Grandma and her other siblings north to Cleveland.

Today, Aunt Laura tells Grandma to grab her coat. Let's go, girl, she says.

They get into Aunt Laura's car and drive to the blue-collar suburb of East Cleveland, which isn't far from the apartment with all the rodents. Aunt Laura and Grandma head down Euclid Avenue, which once had so many stately mansions that it was considered the most beautiful street in the world.

Aunt Laura wheels her car east down Euclid and, after only a few blocks, turns right onto Brightwood Avenue. She drives past a Gulf gas station on the northwest corner of the street and slowly rolls past the first two dwellings, a set of sprawling green apartment buildings and a two-story brown duplex. Aunt Laura pulls into the brick driveway next to the duplex. There sits a white, colonial-style house with red trim.

Baby girl, this house is yours, Aunt Laura says, looking at her younger sister. Grandma believes Aunt Laura must have misspoken. After all Grandma has been through, she can't believe she finally has her own home in a stable neighborhood to raise her seven kids and her grandson.

The house is in my name, Aunt Laura explains, but it's yours. We'll leave it in my name until Queenie gets old enough to put it in her name. You don't want it in your name, Sangenella, because the welfare folks will find out. Just leave it in my name until your daughter turns eighteen and then you can have the name on the deed changed.

Aunt Laura knows how to work the system. She and Grandma get out of the car and go inside the seven-room house. Downstairs is a spacious living room with nice green carpet, a dining room, the master bedroom, a bathroom, and a kitchen. Upstairs are three bedrooms, a den, and a bathroom. There is a large basement with three rooms. The two women walk outdoors and, for the first time, Grandma sees that the backyard has room enough for a garden and a basketball hoop, which will certainly please her three sons. In front, there is a rose bush and a patch of grass big enough to be called a lawn. All this is Grandma's for a five-hundred-dollar down payment and a monthly mortgage of $126.

There are about four dozen frame houses on Brightwood. Most have small yards and sit somewhat close together. But for many of the newest residents, like Grandma, fresh from Cleveland's East-Side ghettos, these homes might as well be mansions. Each home comes with large rooms and solid foundations, driveways and garages. The street itself seems safe and somewhat quiet, yet it is still busy for a residential road.

Brightwood is busy because it is one of the few streets south of Euclid Avenue with its own traffic light. It's an attractive route for far-out suburbanites commuting to jobs downtown or to the nearby University Circle area, home to Lakeside Hospital, Case Western Reserve University, a natural history museum, and a concert hall.

Rush-hour traffic backs up Brightwood from Euclid past our new house, sometimes halfway up the street. We don't see this as an annoyance. It's a chance to see different people and learn about their daily travel routines. The mostly white commuters keep their eyes straight ahead and don't pay much attention to us little kids playing in the yards. Many of these commuters have been coming down Brightwood for years and have watched its social transformation as black families have moved in. They remember how Brightwood used to be. They remember when the parents on the porch and the kids in yards were all white like themselves. They remember how, in just the past year or so, the first black residents started showing up. They have watched over the years, from their cars, as more moving vans become staples on the street, as many whites packed and headed for the outer suburbs. Some of the commuters might even have lived on Brightwood just a few years before.

Even though the commuters know about the transformation of our street and our suburb, they appear not to have been frightened off. Brightwood is a major artery toward points west, and the white commuters continue to travel it, for a while anyway, to get to their well-paying jobs.

I sleep in the middle room on the second floor of our new house. I share the room with my three uncles— Anthony, whom we call Antmo, Bobby, and Bill. They are my mother's three brothers. Antmo is five, Bobby is eight, and Bill is thirteen. Antmo, because of the closeness in our ages, is my best buddy, even though I am only a toddler. While all four of us boys share a bedroom, Antmo and I share a bed. He is a fun playmate, and we do everything together, once he gets home from kindergarten.

Antmo is bigger and rougher than me. I am skin and bones, with no discernible muscles. Antmo is already developing muscles. We also look different. I have a light brownish complexion. My hair is still soft and curly like it was at birth. Antmo is jet black like Leroy, his daddy, and he has woolly hair. He and his daddy are very close. I don't have a daddy around, but my mother is pretty and has a lot of boyfriends who always make a big fuss over me.

I am two and a half in February 1967 when we arrive on Brightwood, so I don't get to go to school, but my sixteen-year-old mother and all the other children do.

I wake up each morning around nine when I hear Grandma's melodic voice calling out for me. If she didn't want my mother having me, you can't tell it now. I seem to be the pride of her life.

Dwayne, honey, time to get up, she says, almost singing as she does every Sunday in the church choir. Yo food's on the table.

I rise and lumber downstairs toward the bathroom. The soap is still wet and slippery from the others who used it before going to school. The toothpaste is uncapped and some has spilled onto the sink counter.

I sit down to a bowl of Cream of Wheat. Grandma has already put sugar in it, too much usually, and some margarine. We can't afford butter. I pour on some Carnation cream, which makes the hot cereal taste special.

I have a red tricycle and, after breakfast, I ride around our new backyard. There are four big cement blocks, and I go from one square to another, as if I'm going from one city to another. I go from Chicago to New York to Cleveland. I don't know about any other places in the world, so I confine my game to those northern cities, towns where I've heard grown-ups say there is plenty of opportunity for blacks.

Grandma is in the kitchen washing dishes, and I can see the dish towel in her hand as she talks to me through the crack in the raised window. Leroy, Grandma's boyfriend who is going to marry her one day, is still asleep. He snores loudly. He works six days a week from 4:30 P.M. to 1:00 A.M. at a Jewish restaurant in suburban South Euclid. When he gets home from work, he watches television until all the stations sign off with a loud beeping sound. If you wake up early enough, sometimes the television is still on and nothing but static is on the screen. Other times, Leroy lies there sleeping and the TV station signs back on before he awakens.

Sometimes Grandma takes me to the strip shopping center eight blocks from our house. We go in and out of the shops and, at the supermarket, Grandma purchases groceries. We walk back down Euclid Avenue toward Brightwood.

When Grandma is shopping for a lot of groceries, we never walk because there are too many bags. Then, she says, Wake up yo Granddaddy, meaning Leroy, who is really not my grandfather. My grandfather is Samuel Bray and he lives down south somewhere.

I rouse Leroy from his sleep and we get into his 1961 Buick Wildcat, a gold car that Leroy prides more than anything else. We drive to the shopping center or downtown to the West Side Market, where there are a bunch of fruit, vegetable, and meat stands. But you have to bring your own shopping bags.

By fall, a lot of teenage boys come around to our house every evening on school days and the weekends. They are there to see my mother, who is seventeen, and her younger sister Pat, who is four months shy of her sixteenth birthday. I'm not sure why they call her Pat because her given name is Aletha, but I call her that, too. I later understand why all those boys are hanging around our house. Within months, Pat is pregnant. Grandma is upset all right. She already is helping raise me, and now another grandchild is on the way.

Pat's boyfriend is named Calvin, and he's from a street right off St. Clair Avenue in Cleveland. St. Clair, along with Euclid and Superior, are the three major thoroughfares on the East Side of Cleveland. Calvin is a flashy dresser who works at some factory as a laborer. He has a nasal voice and comes in the house and greets everybody with a hug and kiss. He likes movies about the Mafia. Grandma likes him because he seems to have money all the time and he is country. When she calls his name, Calvin answers, Yes, ma'am. She likes that, too. It reminds her of the boys in Cecil, not these disrespectful boys in the big city. Of course, Grandma doesn't think it's good form to turn away a man who is kind and showers us with money.

I like Calvin a lot and wish he were my father. Sometimes, he treats me like I'm his son. He has a friend named Coochie, whom everybody is trying to fix up with my mother. Coochie is not cool like Calvin. Sometimes, my mother and Pat and Calvin and Coochie go out on dates together in Calvin's car. Calvin has a big Cadillac that's about eight years old, but he says he's going to get a new, better car that will be the talk of the town.

Pat's stomach gets bigger, and on November 13, 1969, she goes to Booth Memorial Hospital, where she delivers the baby. Like his father, the baby's name is Calvin. Now we call them Big Calvin and Little Calvin.

The day after Little Calvin is born, my mother takes me to the hospital to see my first cousin for the first time. There is a lot of whispering in the waiting room about whether Big Calvin can visit Pat and the baby because Pat is an unwed mother and the welfare department and Booth Hospital do not want Calvin visiting. If the father doesn't own up to being the father and pay the medical bill, he isn't recognized by the state. I can't understand why the welfare people hate men so much. I wonder if the caseworkers will hate me, too, when I'm grown. I also can't understand why the welfare department has to pay for Pat to have this baby, because I know that Big Calvin has more money than the welfare department and the state of Ohio combined.

Little Calvin is in the nursery with a bunch of other babies. He is long and skinny with really light skin and a head full of curly hair. He will be coming home to our house on Brightwood soon. But he is too small to sleep in the room with the rest of us boys, so he will sleep in the room with my mother and his mother.

Life for me doesn't change much when Little Calvin comes home from the hospital, even though at five years old I'm no longer the baby of the family. Little Calvin is so skinny that Leroy starts calling him Wiener. I think everyone adapts to the nickname so well because they were already getting tired of distinguishing between Big Calvin and Little Calvin.

By the time of Wiener's birth in 1969, the only whites left on our street are elderly women who are either too set in their ways to move or perhaps can't afford to.

Grandma doesn't care that the whites are all moving out. We were only the third or fourth black family to move onto Brightwood. But now, not even three years later, only about a half dozen of the homes are occupied by white families. And none of those are families with children. Grandma loves East Cleveland. The city picks up the rubbish twice a week and the public schools have a reputation for excellence. East Cleveland also has active church groups, well-stocked libraries, a mom-and-pop store in every neighborhood, and its very own regional train and bus station.

Not far from our house is Forest Hills Park, a beautiful fifty-acre park on land donated to East Cleveland and neighboring Cleveland Heights by the late oil tycoon, John D. Rockefeller. A century earlier, Rockefeller had bought 109 acres of land and built an opulent house there. He and his family lived in East Cleveland for thirty-five years until a dispute with tax authorities forced him to move to New York. He only came back after his death, to be buried in nearby Lakeview Cemetery on his old property.

Most of the black families moving into East Cleveland are hard-working people who are only looking for a better way of life. The people who move to Brightwood are no different. By 1970, residents of the street form a block club that organizes monthly street cleanups. The work isn't hard because there are so many helping hands. Kool-Aid, cookies, and potato chips are served, and by late afternoon the committee starts the cookout. Everybody takes so much pride in our neighborhood to show we can keep it just as clean as the white folks had.

◪ Two ◪

It's late summer of 1970, and I'm already excited about starting kindergarten in a couple of weeks. But one afternoon Grandma grabs my spotlight by announcing that she and Leroy are getting married.

Antmo starts jumping up and down and throwing his hands in the air like he has just scored the winning touchdown in a big football game. He is screaming, Yeah! Yeah! Yeah! I hadn't known that he even cared his parents weren't married.

As he is jumping around the room, he gets a foot caught in the legs of a chair, and his body comes crashing toward a coffee table. He lands face first. His lip is busted, and about 25 percent of one front tooth is chipped away. He is messed up, but he's still happy that Grandma is getting married.

It won't be easy, because Grandma and Leroy are both already married. Grandma is still married to her second husband, William Brimage, and Leroy is still married to his first wife, whom I don't know. Grandma and Leroy were both separated from their spouses when they met, and neither had any intentions of rekindling those relationships. The problem is that Leroy has a fourth-grade education and Grandma has a tenth-grade one from a Jim Crow school system, which means it is inferior. That's why both of them have such a hard time figuring out how to navigate the system, why neither one has figured out how to get their divorces finalized.

When Grandma and her first husband, Sam Bray, divorced, he and his family handled everything. But this time she has to file the papers to divorce Brimage. She finally gets it done on June 23, but the question is, will the divorce of Leroy and his wife be final by September 18, the day of the wedding? Antmo's birthday is September 17, so he expects the wedding as his birthday gift, if his father can get the legal work done in time.

Meanwhile, my first day of school is approaching and my mother has to get me a fresh haircut. She can do special things for me now because she has finished high school and has a secretarial job as a unit clerk at St. Vincent Charity Hospital.

◨

Since she is working, I believe she and I are off welfare, unless Grandma still collects it for some reason. I don't know and I don't ask. I know my mother used to argue with Grandma all the time about how she spends the money the welfare department gives her for my care. She used to say Grandma didn't buy me any good clothes, and Grandma told her that the clothes she gets from the Goodwill are good enough for her own children and they are good enough for me. One day my mother gets so fed up with Grandma's refusal to spend money on some new shoes for me that she goes out and tries to steal me a pair from Woolworth's. She gets arrested.

Now that she's high school–educated and working, she can afford to buy me things, especially since we live with Grandma and don't have any big rent or mortgage. And a special haircut is one of those things.

Dexter is our neighborhood barber, and he cuts the hair of Leroy, Bill, Bobby, and Antmo. But my mother thinks my hair is too good for any old barber, so she wants to take me to Cooke's Barber Shop on the corner of Lakeview and Superior. She says they are stylists.

Since we don't own a car, my mother and I walk several miles to the barber shop. She smokes Kool cigarettes. She is wearing a short brown skirt that stops high above her knees. Men like to look at those legs, but I just think they are too long because she walks so fast I can hardly keep up with her. I want her to slow down but she doesn't. She calls out for me to walk faster. She smokes and walks, and I run to try to keep up.

Finally, we make it to Cooke's, but Mr. Cooke is nowhere to be found. My mother lets someone else cut my hair. He's no better than Dexter.

◻

My mother's getting dressed to go somewhere. I can tell by how much attention she is paying to her lipstick and other makeup. She says her boyfriend, Billy, is picking her up.

Ooh, I wanna go.

No, not this time.

Why not?

'Cause, you can't.

Within no time, a black Fleetwood rolls into our red-brick driveway. Billy's car has a vanity tire in the back. It's a four-door with black leather seats. Inside is an eight-track tape player. The steering wheel is covered with leather. Billy, very tall and slender, gets out, dressed in black leather pants. His pants match his pitch-black skin and his hair is cut in a short Afro. He has on expensive jewelry, nothing gaudy, but rich. He has a male friend with him.

Antmo and several other kids run over to this cool car, like the kind we see in the movies on TV. Someone asks, Hey Dwayne, is that yo daddy? I don't answer; I want them to think that it is. Who wouldn't want a daddy with this bad ride?

Billy climbs our front steps, walks onto the porch, and takes a seat on our thin wooden rail banisters. His buddy sits next to him.

Watch this, he says to his friend. Hey, Dwayne? What you wanna be when you grow up?

I say the only thing I can think of—a basketball player in the NBA and, if I can't be that, I'll be a doctor or a lawyer. A big smile creases my face. But Billy looks crestfallen.

Nah, man, that ain't how you make money, he says. I'm going to ask you again, now give me the right answer. His friend is watching intently, waiting for the right answer.

Billy again asks, Hey, Dwayne, what you wanna be when you get big?

I look at Billy and I blurt out, A pimp!

Billy and his friend laugh and slap five. That's my cat, Billy says in a slow deep voice. That's my cat. This little motherfucker gonna tear this city up when he get big. He's gonna have all the women.

He reaches in his pocket and slips me some coins.

I normally cry when my mother leaves without me. After she and Billy and the other man pull off, Antmo walks over.

How much you got? my seven-year-old uncle asks.

I pull out my coins. Fifty cents, I say.

Antmo and I dash to the corner, cross Euclid, and go to the A&A Suprette for some candy.

◪

Everybody is getting ready for the wedding. But Leroy, four days prior to it, is still not divorced from his first wife. The lawyers finally get everything taken care of, and on September 15 he is officially divorced. Three days later, in our living room on Brightwood, Grandma and

Leroy tie the knot in a service officiated by our pastor, Reverend Lee James Jones. Calvin and I sit next to each other. Our mothers and their brothers and sisters are all there. And so are all of Grandma's sisters and brothers who live in Cleveland—Aunts Laura, Bessie, Willa, and Dorothy and Uncles Columbus and Adell. I meet new cousins, and after the wedding there is a reception right there at the house. The music is loud and everybody dances until around 10 P.M., when they make Antmo and me go upstairs and away from the party. Grandma and Leroy hug and kiss and seem happy.

One Saturday before the fall of 1970, I am helping Antmo and Dent, our friend from up the street, build a hot rod that we have been working on for several days. We have wheels from an old, broken-down wagon, some two-by-fours, string for a hand-held steering wheel, and some paint for design. We are working and working, mostly Antmo and Dent, but at least I am staying out of their way. The two older boys leave me alone and head out of our garage. They return with Sharlene, a neighborhood girl who is considered a tomboy because she plays rough and has short hair.

There is an old refrigerator in our garage. Sharlene leans against it and we press our bodies against hers, one at a time. She unbuttons her shirt and reveals a flat chest that is no different from any of ours. We take turns feeling Sharlene's chest and sticking our hands down her pants and rubbing our bodies against hers. This goes on for only a few minutes before Sharlene leaves.

For me, the incident is remarkable and the wheels in my six-year-old head start spinning. Maybe I can do this with her when Dent and Antmo aren't around, I think.

So that same evening, before sundown, I am playing in the yard and Sharlene appears out of nowhere. We are normal playing partners but now, because of the earlier incident, our relationship has some new context. I ask her into the garage next to the old fridge with me. She complies and I press my lips together and kiss her. I am trying to pull down her pants but as soon as I get them unbuttoned, into the garage walks Leroy, Grandma's husband. What y'all doin'? he asks. Sharlene fastens her pants and runs out of the garage.

Nuthin', I claim.

I'm gonna tell yo grandma, he says.

The reaction of everybody is strange. I don't get into any real trouble. No one tells me what I had been doing with Sharlene is wrong. Instead, I get tagged as being sweet on a girl who everybody considers to be a tomboy. Even Antmo and Dent laugh at me, but I never tell the adults that Antmo and Dent are the ones who taught me to go in the garage and behind the refrigerator with Sharlene.

The turf disputes and violence that many black families on our street had known in the ghettos of Cleveland follow us to East Cleveland. Just a few years after our arrival, Brightwood has become like an oasis unto itself for the residents of this street. The people who live here, especially the teenagers and younger children, have adopted an attitude that we are superior to other youngsters on neighboring streets. Brightwood develops a dislike for its neighbor to the west, Penrose, and vice versa.

One early evening during the summer of 1971, the smell of chicken from the Red Barn, a restaurant on the corner of nearby Wadena, is wafting through our neighborhood. I am playing in the yard with Antmo when gunfire rings out in the distance, *bam-bam-bam*.

Y'all get y'all's asses in the house! My mother's sister Marie screams out, running on the porch to see where we are. Bobby, Antmo, and I run in the house.

They are at it again—the older boys and some men on Brightwood and Penrose are fighting, and this time, they're shooting.

Marie tells us to stay down. All of a sudden, Grandma appears. She's in a panic and asks, Where's Bill?

The answer, of course, is that Bill, now sixteen, is probably not far from the shooting. He runs with a pack of young rowdies from the street. There is Ron Veasley, who doesn't take much off anyone, and Terry and Larry Veasley, both a little older and more mature than Ron and Bill. But Terry and Larry are tough as well, so I wouldn't doubt that they are near the shooting, too.

One of the older Dent boys, Michael, has to be involved if Bill and the Veasleys are, that's for sure. So no doubt up at the Dent household, my friends Pokey and Dent are on their knees staying out of the way of gunfire, just like Antmo and me. And their mother is saying, Where's Michael?

This standoff lasts into the summer night, and we are not allowed to go outside. Whenever one of the older children, such as my mother or Pat, makes it home, they report that the police have set up a command post at each corner of Brightwood and Penrose and are checking identification before letting residents enter either street. They say the cops are scared to come down either street; that's why they have set up their command posts on the corners. I don't blame the cops. I am thinking, These niggas are crazy. They'll kill anyone.

But mostly I'm thinking about Bill. What if he gets shot and killed? Who will let me sit on his back when we are watching television, and who will bring me stolen toys home after school?

The crisis ends with no fatalities on either side. I am told that one Penrose guy was shot and others on both streets beaten.

Bill returns home, but I never find out where he had been. For several weeks, I'm urged not to go to the A&A Suprette. Those dudes on Penrose might catch you and beat you or even kill you, someone would say. My mother confines me to Brightwood, close to our house at all times.

⬛

By early 1972, Bobby, Antmo, and I live for Friday nights. Calvin, not yet two, is too little to stay up very late. But this is Leroy's night off. Early in the day, Bobby, Antmo, and I go to the corner store and buy a bag of popcorn seeds for thirty-nine cents. We keep it for nighttime. Leroy helps us set up pallets on the living room floor. We pop the corn and then melt a half stick of margarine and pour it over the popcorn. We then sit in the living room and watch television shows, such as *The Avengers* with Emma Peel. After that, we watch the *Hoolihan and Big Chuck Show*. The hosts are two local celebrities who show a movie and do skits between commercials. Sometimes Bill will join us, if he gets home in time. Many nights he stays out late. When he's watching television with us, he stretches out on the floor in front of the television and I climb on his back. He is getting taller, maybe he's six foot two now and he's still just seventeen. These nights of watching television with Leroy, Bill, Bobby, and Antmo are some of the best nights of my life, if the popcorn isn't burnt.

⬚

I am still the best dresser in my second-grade class. I frequently wear an expensive suit, a maxilength coat, and a tam. I am lucky, I believe, to have the youngest mother in the history of the second grade who is so fashion-conscious that she spends outrageous sums of money on my clothes and upkeep. My teacher dotes on me. I seem to be a poster child for everything that is right in the working-class suburb of East Cleveland. We are all well groomed and fairly smart. Look at us and you believe little black kids can achieve as well as those white kids in the suburbs.

⬚

My mother lives with her boyfriend, Murray Tyson, and I stay with them a lot. Murray lives in an apartment on Hayden Avenue right outside the East Cleveland border. I like Murray's place. Not only do I get the television to myself to watch sports all weekend, but Murray's apartment is neat and clean and full of pricey furniture and electronic equipment, just the opposite of the house on Brightwood with all my aunts and uncles and my cousin Little Calvin. There are plants and flowers and sweet-smelling stuff. Murray's big color TV sits in a living room with wood panel floors. His tables all have rugs under them. His couch and chairs are all soft black leather. He has interesting artwork on the wall, and a great collection of albums and eight-track tapes to play on his hi-fi stereo system. He likes to listen to jazz.

He keeps plenty of food in the refrigerator, and not just leftovers. He has all types of cheese and deli meat and lots of fruit. On Brightwood, Grandma's only concern is feeding us breakfast and dinner. Lunch is hit-and-miss there. Most of the food she prepares is designed to merely keep us going. It's not cuisine. She has too little money and too many kids and grandkids to feed for it to be any other way.

At Murray's, it is only him, my mother, and I. We eat three square meals a day, including lunch. There are snacks at night during the prime-time television hour. For dinner, we might have T-bone steaks with mashed potatoes and gravy and wheat bread. It is always wheat bread, which I really don't like, but I never say so because I'm grateful. Corned beef sandwiches and salad are lunchtime fare. Breakfast consists of pancakes with Mrs. Butterworth's syrup and sausages. At Grandma's, we always have the cheaper Alaga brand syrup.

◪

It's Friday, October 6, 1972. Before Antmo and I can get out of bed, Grandma is in our room telling us to get up. Y'all ain't going to school today. Yo Aunt Laura died overnight, she says.

I am sad that Aunt Laura is dead. I know she has done a lot for us, even though I don't know the specifics. I enjoy going over to her house in Cleveland. To get there, you have to go up a hill, and there are pears in her back-yard that we always pick. Sometimes she would holler out the window for us to get out of the tree, and other times she would tell us to get a bag and go in the back and pick some pears to take home. We would eat pears all night, until we didn't want to see any more of them.

Aunt Laura had a reputation for being mean. She had gotten shot years earlier when a man tried to gun down her younger brother, Adell. She stepped in front of Adell and took the bullet for him, everybody says. Her face was partly disfigured because she had a skin graft after the shooting. She always told me I was going to be smart and make something out of myself one day because I am curious. That gave me confidence to get mostly As in school. But now she's dead.

Not only did Aunt Laura get us the house on Brightwood and take care of Grandma after their own mother died, she also brought Grandma to Cleveland and showed her how to take care of her money and spend it wisely. Perhaps that's why Grandma always buys clothes from the Goodwill. Aunt Laura also adopted two kids, Skipper and Marva, whom Bobby, Antmo, and I played with when we went over to her house.

Grandma leaves the room and I ask Antmo if he knows anyone else who is dead. He says I should quit asking so many damn questions, just like that, he says it. I am always asking questions and I don't know why I ask Antmo. He never has the answer. I'll soon be eight and he's ten and it seems like I have more answers to things than he does. But I like him anyway. He's fun. Having him around is like having an older brother who will play with you.

That morning, everybody is moving with purposeful intent. Grandma is on the phone, talking to business folks all morning—the hospital, the insurance company, and the funeral home. Grandma is sad. Her mother died at forty, and now her favorite sister is gone at forty-one. Both had cancer. Grandma is wondering why God chose to take away at an early age these two women she has counted on most in her own thirty-nine years on this earth. Surely, if it hadn't been for Aunt Laura, Grandma might still be stuck in Cecil. And she definitely wouldn't have this four-bedroom house. And Grandma is also thinking whether she will live past her early forties or die like her mother and sister.

While Grandma is on the phone, Antmo and I grab a bag of Wheat Puff cereal off the top of the fridge. We keep it there so the mice and rats won't get to it. I pour some cereal in a bowl, sprinkle on some sugar, and pour in the milk. Grandma is sitting in a chair away from the kitchen table and talking to the hospital about Aunt Laura. Pretty soon, she and Leroy get in the car and leave.

Antmo, Bobby, and I stay home with Marie, who is saying she is not going to Aunt Laura's funeral because when you're pregnant your baby will be born disfigured if you go to a funeral. It doesn't make sense to me. Marie, like my mother and Pat before her, is an unwed teenage-mother-to-be. Marie is sixteen. Why would your baby be messed up if you go to a funeral? I ask her.

She thinks for a while and then gets irritated. Quit asking so many damn questions, she says, just like Antmo. You always got questions to ask, Dwayne. You just don't go to funerals when you're pregnant. Everybody knows that. Now go outside.

This is my first funeral, and I'm afraid because I've never seen a dead person before. I don't know what to do or how I'm supposed to act. It is warm inside the funeral parlor on this crisp October day in 1972. Mama and her other sisters are sitting in the first row, while we sit further back. Mama cries, but Aunt Bessie shouts louder than everyone. She throws her arms in the air and starts saying, Baby, baby, baby! What are we going to do without you? My sister, please, baby don't leave us. Laura, Laura.

Aunt Bessie is in front of the aisle, near the casket, and ushers rush over to assist her.

I try to force myself to cry because crying seems to be

the right thing to do. Everyone there is crying but me. But try as I might, the tears won't come, so I sit there next to Antmo, wondering why I can't cry because I do love Aunt Laura. Soon it is my row's turn to walk past the body. The casket is about as blue as the sky on a clear Cleveland summer day. The interior is white, and there is a lot of padding. The body fits right in the middle of this skinny box, without much room to spare. I wonder what happens if you die, but then wake up after the casket is shut. Do they lock caskets? I think, When I die I don't want the casket locked, in case I turn out not to be really dead.

Aunt Laura looks like herself. She seems content, at peace. She lies there, her eyes shut, and I stop and study her.

The body is placed in a hearse, and the procession heads toward our neighborhood to Lakeview Cemetery. Even at the funeral home, many of the mourners had already started to make a big deal out of the fact that Aunt Laura will be buried on the same land as John D. Rockefeller. Once the procession is inside the gates, the cemetery seems to never end and the procession goes around winding roads for a long time before we come to Aunt Laura's burial plot. The smell of roses fills the air. The Reverend Jones says a few words of prayer at the cemetery, and we all get back in our cars and go home, just five blocks away.

At home, I go upstairs and take off my suit and tie. I'm up here by myself in the back room, hanging up my suit, and I hear a noise in the closet.

No, Aunt Laura! I scream, dashing out of the room and down the stairs. Don't get me! Grandma tells me Aunt Laura is not going to hurt me, that she's gone to Heaven for all the great things she's done, including helping us get this house. I feel better and go back upstairs to face my demons, alone.

◪

After Aunt Laura's death, one of Grandma's brothers starts living with us. His name is Columbus Williams, but for some reason we all call him Uncle Son. He picked up the nickname Son in Cecil, Alabama, and all I can guess is it's because he was his father's first biological son after five girls: Bessie, Sangenella, Laura, Dorothy, and Willa.

Uncle Son is a sweet and gentle man. He has short-cropped black hair and is about five foot nine. He weighs around 180 pounds, but has strength that belies his dimensions. People say he's so strong because he grew up on a farm, and that farm boys are supposed to be strong, unlike city boys who, I guess, are supposed to be weak.

Unc collects a disability check each month because he can't work regular hours. He is on a prescription medicine called Thorazine, but he sometime fails to take it. That's when he acts weird. Like Leroy, he snores at night. Sometime Unc wakes up in the middle of a bad dream, screaming DADDY! DADDY! DADDY! or JOHN HALL! JOHN HALL! JOHN HALL! Grandma tells us that John Hall is the man who ran the general store in Cecil when they were youngsters. I don't know why Unc is so afraid of John Hall. Grandma, however, says John Hall was a nice old white man who was fair to blacks in Cecil.

Sometimes Unc shouts for his late sister, my Aunt Laura, whose full name was Laura Bell Williams. LAURA B! LAURA B! LAURA B! Grandma says we kids should pay Unc no mind. The older kids in the house, my mother's sisters and brothers, call Unc crazy and say a tree fell on Unc's head when he was kid. He hasn't been the same since, if you listen to them. It's funny living in a house with your Grandma's brother, who is your great-uncle, and all your mother's sisters and brothers, who are your aunts and uncles. Only great-uncles and great-aunts get the respect of really being your elders. My mother's siblings are more like my own brothers and sisters, only older. But not that much older.

Whenever Unc's condition gets too bad, Grandma and Leroy drive him to Fairhill or Hawthorne hospitals, which my mother's sisters and brothers tell me are for crazy people. I find it strange because when I go with Grandma to take Unc some cigarettes and money for the commissary, Fairhill and Hawthorne both seem like nice quiet places. Everybody is calm, far more calm than the folks with whom I live. But Unc resists being taken away most times. That's when Grandma phones the East Cleveland police. Officers come and place him in handcuffs and wrestle with him until they can force him into the back of the squad car. If he gets too violent, they'll take him to jail, which upsets Grandma because she says he's sick, not criminal. I find that strange, too, because she is the one who calls the police on him in the first place.

After a week or two away, Unc usually comes back to our home and takes his medication regularly.

Unc, to me, is harmless, despite his enormous strength. I've never seen him hurt anyone, even when he fights with the police officers. When his disability check arrives or when he gets paid under the table from his occasional work at a local car wash, he gives money to all us kids. Having him around is like having another kid in the house, one who has the privileges and the freedom of a grown person.

Unc is old enough to buy beer and wine from A&A Suprette. Sometime he gets so drunk that the owner,

Mr. Horne, will refuse to sell to him. Mama has told Mr. Horne and other owners of stores in the area that if they sell him too much and he gets hit by a car crossing Euclid Avenue, she's going to sue them. Still, no matter how drunk he gets, Unc never gets hit by the cars that speed up and down the busy main street.

Bobby, Antmo, and I steal money from Unc all the time. We reason that if we steal his money, he'll have less with which to buy alcohol. He stashes his money under the mattress on his small twin bed with the soft, white leather headboard. When he goes to sleep, one of us crawls beside his bed and swipes a few dollars from his billfold, especially during the first part of the month when his disability check, in the dark yellow envelope, arrives. Because Unc is usually drunk and snoring loudly, he doesn't wake up when he is being robbed. By the time he sobers up and notices the missing cash, we have already spent it on candy and pop.

With Unc, our house is becoming overcrowded, especially since he isn't the only new addition to the family. Pat and Wayne Carter, the man she married several months before Aunt Laura's funeral, are now living with us as well.

Wayne is from the housing projects not far from downtown. He and Pat met five years earlier when Wayne lived in East Cleveland and quarterbacked the Shaw High football team. Pat was a Shaw High cheerleader at the time. Wayne eventually got into trouble, was sent to a home for unruly boys in Columbus, and Pat wound up having a baby by Big Calvin.

Pat always liked Wayne. Unlike Big Calvin, he isn't flashy and his presence doesn't intimidate her as much.

My mother is living with Murray, and Little Calvin and I sleep in the green bunk beds in the same second-floor room with the newlyweds, who have a queen-sized bed. Pat and Wayne's marriage is off to a rocky start and they argue much of the time, especially at night when I'm trying to sleep. Sometimes, he hits and slaps her. I pretend to be asleep, but I hear all of this. I am glad when I hear Grandma's voice calling from downstairs.

Pat? Wayne? Why y'all keeping up all that fuss?

I'm trying to sleep, Mrs. Brimage, but she won't let me. She keeps arguin', Wayne says. He doesn't mention that he hit her.

Pat, leave that boy alone, Grandma says to her eighteen-year-old, married daughter.

I wonder if they know I'm awake. I try to be as still as possible in this top bunk so they won't suspect I hear their fight. But who can't hear them? I wonder if Little Calvin is awake, but he doesn't move either. Amazingly, he appears to be sound asleep. He's just turned three, five years younger than me.

Eventually Pat, Wayne, and Little Calvin get their own apartment in the Outhwaite Homes Public Housing Projects, near East Fifty-fifth Street. Wayne's family lives not far from Outhwaite in another portion of the projects, one with a reputation for toughness. Wayne has two younger sisters, Angie and Gina; two older ones, Cookie and Tissie; and an older brother, Donnie. I get to meet all his sisters, but I never meet Donnie, who is reputed to be the toughest of the Carter clan. When I go down to Outhwaite to visit, I'm told Donnie is in prison after having to kill someone. That's how it's put, *having* to kill the person, as if it was kill or be killed. I don't ask too many questions and just accept his status for what it is.

I am disappointed that Calvin is moving to the projects.

With Calvin, Antmo, and Bobby in the house, I don't need a lot of friends outside it. On rainy or snowy days, we have enough boys in our own family to play whatever games we can think of. Pat senses I'm sad and says I can visit her and Calvin in the projects any weekend. I'm not sure I want Pat living with Wayne because they seem to fight all the time. Also, Wayne is known for attracting violence. Some man shot Wayne shortly after they got married. It happened when Pat and Wayne were walking down Central Avenue in the housing projects where Wayne's family lives. The man jumped out of a car with a pistol in his hand, asked Wayne if he had the money the man accused Wayne of owing him. Wayne told the man he didn't owe him anything, and the man shot Wayne in the neck and arm and then stared at Pat, who ran like hell. The man jumped in his car and left, and Pat ended up going to Mississippi for a while until things settled down. Wayne stayed in the hospital for weeks and hasn't worked since because his injuries were disabling. I fear for Calvin's safety.

One day in the spring of 1973, a bunch of us boys from Brightwood are playing tackle football with some boys from Wadena because they are our friends, unlike the boys from Penrose, who are our enemies.

The playground, which sits behind Mo's gas station, has a merry-go-round, sliding board, and swing set. There is also a grassy area about forty yards long and twenty yards wide that we use to play football.

Antmo catches a little flare pass and is running for a touchdown, but he is tackled about five yards short of the goal line. The ball scoots out of his grasp. Not knowing if it is a fumble, I pick up the ball and head the other way.

Antmo gives chase and starts to gain on me. I am nearing my goal line for a touchdown when Antmo catches me from behind and drives my little nine-year-old body into the ground. On the way down, my left knee gets caught under a rusty muffler the men at Mo's have thrown out behind the gas station. The sharp end of the muffler tears through my jeans and into my kneecap. Blood soils my jeans above my knee. I holler out. Someone lifts up my pant leg and flesh is hanging out above my knee.

David Hairston, who is about four years older and twice my size, picks me up and carries me home. Grandma says, Oh, my baby. How did this happen to him?

Someone says Antmo tackled me and Grandma doesn't understand the word tackle, as in, we were playing a game. She threatens to give Antmo the worst whipping he's ever had. Oh, my baby, she keeps saying.

She doesn't believe too much in doctors and, anyway, she has too many children and grandchildren and sees too many injuries to run to the hospital every time an old rusty muffler slices open someone's knee. So, she pours some peroxide on the wound.

I hobble around school on my bad knee after the injury. One day we are lining up for lunch, and I can barely move because my knee is throbbing. I am not moving fast enough for Greg Horn and he pushes me and says, Hurry up! My knee turns slightly and starts to bleed.

I don't like him pushing me because I am from Brightwood and don't take any crap off any other second grader. So I push Greg back, and we agree to settle our differences after school. Normally I believe I can whip Greg, but this bum knee is going to present a problem.

After school, I am leaving the building and out of nowhere somebody grabs me from behind. It is Greg's brother, who is a fifth grader. Greg and his brother are new at school, and they do not realize that they are not supposed to mess with kids from Brightwood and neighboring Wadena. They come from a tough city school and think the kids in East Cleveland are soft, especially a scrawny second grader like myself.

Greg's brother has me in a full bear hug and Greg is punching me all over, in the chest, face, and body. A crowd forms and everybody is screaming, Fight! Fight! Fight! Greg kicks me square in my injured knee and laughs. You don't look so tough now, he taunts.

My knee is bleeding and the dark red blood is soaking through the leg of my pants. Greg's brother lets go of me finally. They call me names and walk off laughing.

I am in pain and crying like a baby, something I never do in front of my classmates. I hobble over to the old red-brick building that houses the upper grades at Superior, looking for Antmo, Dent, and the older boys from Brightwood and Wadena. Finally, I bump into Slate, a fifth grader who lives on Wadena and sometimes hangs around with Antmo and Dent. Slate is tall and has hands as large as a tenth grader's. He says he knows where Dent, Antmo, and Chuck Veasley are. Chuck is tough, too—a thick fifth grader who knows how to fight well and isn't afraid of anybody. We find them, and, sobbing, I tell them my story.

Slate says, Let's go find their asses.

They all run down Garfield Avenue to Euclid. I hobble behind. On Euclid, Slate catches up with the Horn boys. He holds Greg and his older brother until I catch up and make a positive identification. As soon as I say, He's the one who had me in the bear hug, pointing to Greg's older brother, Slate rears back with those big, high-school hands and pops him dead in the nose. I can hear the sounds of cartilage breaking under the weight of the heavy punch.

Blood pours out and Greg's brother is begging Slate to stop, but by then all the other boys are jumping on Greg's brother, too. I run over to Greg and start hitting him in the face. He recoils, as if he wants to fight back, but with a half dozen menacing, bigger boys from my street staring him down, he takes my beating without a fight.

I am so happy, so proud to be from Brightwood.

The next day we are all called into the school office. We tell Mr. Adams, the principal, our version of what transpired, how the Horns first attacked me. He finds us responsible. He says I should have reported the Horn boys to the office, not sought out my own revenge. Mr. Adams says he's decided our punishment will be five swats apiece with his paddle, a short piece of taped-up wood he keeps in his office. When my turn comes for the paddling, I am crying before he even hits me. Mr. Adams pulls up my pants so they are tight around my buttocks, makes me bend over, and swats me. It stings so badly and I cry so loudly that he decides to give me only two swats, three fewer than the bigger boys. We are lectured and all given passes to return to class. In the hallway, the others who have been pretending to cry start laughing. I am the only one shedding real tears.

◩ Three ◩

My mother has been gone for months. She calls occasionally. She is in Toronto. I know Canada is on the other side of Lake Erie, where Grandma and Leroy take me fishing. When we go to the lake, sometime I just stand on the big rocks that stretch out into the water and pray to God that my mother will come back to Cleveland and take me with her wherever she goes. But

God doesn't seem to be listening.

My mother misses my ninth birthday, October 18, 1973. I am disappointed, but she phones from Toronto. What are you doing there? I demand. She doesn't really answer, and tells me Grandma will take good care of me. My problem is that my mother has spoiled me. She used to give me the best clothes and take me out to dinner and to the circus and carnival. Now she's gone, and Grandma treats me like she treats her own boys. We get only the basics and I am not adjusting well to this change in lifestyle.

Happy birthday, Dwayne, she says over the phone. I will be home soon and will bring you the greatest gift you've ever had.

Several weeks later, as I walk through the giant parking lot of the Red Barn restaurant with some friends, I see my mother standing on our porch. A white Eldorado with white leather seats is parked in the driveway. It belongs to Curtis Walker, her newest boyfriend, the man with whom she went to Canada.

I run toward her, but before I can get there, I see a shiny new bike out of the corner of my eyes. Her arms are out, waiting to embrace me, but I run for the bike instead.

Dwayne! she yells. You betta give me a hug first.

Oh, yeah, I say. I run and give her an obligatory embrace. And then I take the bike, a red Schwinn three-speed, pull it down the stairs, and pedal up the block.

Days later, we are sitting on the porch and I can tell my mother wants to say something important. She just keeps staring at me.

I'm going to Atlanta with Curtis, she says.

I'm going, I say.

Dwayne, you need to be here, in one place, she says. I won't always be at home. You need to stay here with Mama.

Why can't I go? I ask. You never take me with you.

Why won't you take me with you?

My mother is twenty-three and Curtis is at least thirty-five, with an already graying beard. He wears wire-rimmed glasses and has a smooth demeanor, always calm. His style of dress is more low-key than Big Calvin's, but his clothes seem to be even more expensive. He wears gold chains, not very big ones, just ones that look like they cost a bunch of money. His shirts are often silk and his slacks, too. His shoes are leather and perhaps alligator, which is a big thing in our community. Anyone who wears 'gator shoes has got it going on. I don't like him as much as Murray, but that's probably because since he came into the picture my mother is always on the road.

◣

I don't know what happened, but my mother tells me several days later that I can go to Atlanta with her and Curtis. We get into his Eldorado one day and head south on Interstate 71. On the way out of Cleveland, I see a big billboard on the highway touting a local television program called *Morning Exchange* on Channel 5, the ABC affiliate. I wave goodbye to the picture of Fred Griffith, one of the cohosts. Before I started school, I used to watch that show every morning by myself, while waiting for 9 A.M. and *Sesame Street.*

Our car passes the cornfields of rural Ohio in Medina and Ashland counties. I read the signs and count off the miles to the next big city. Finally, after nearly two and one-half hours, we make it to the state capital, Columbus. We put more gas in the car and head over to Cincinnati, where we pick up a different highway, Interstate 75. After another seven hours, we're in Atlanta, the capital of the south, as people call it.

You'll like this place, my mother says. She's talking about the hotel we stay in for our first week in Atlanta. We eventually land in a townhouse in suburban East Point. I like the area. It is a step up from East Cleveland, more like the suburbs in far-out Cleveland where all the white folks from Brightwood moved after our arrival. Our townhouse is fairly new, with two levels and a lot of space. Actually, it turns out to be more spacious than we need. All the space is mostly for me, because I am about to spend a lot of time at home alone.

I gotta go to Miami, Dwayne, my mother suddenly announces one day. She asks me for one favor.

If Grandma calls, tell her I'm at work at Southern Bell.

I do not quite understand why I have to tell my grandmother that my mother works at the phone company when, in fact, she does not. I know she doesn't work there, and she knows she doesn't work there, but I'm supposed to make Grandma believe she works there?

My mother calls when she gets to Miami.

I hope to be home this week, she says.

She doesn't make it. It's Curtis and me. We have never before spent any real time together, but now is our chance to make up for lost time. The only problem is, most nights Curtis isn't home either until very late, if at all. Which means that at age nine, I'm left alone six hundred miles away from Brightwood. Curtis doesn't have a regular job, but he has big wads of cash all the time.

◩

It's night outside and storming, My mother is in Miami, and Curtis is out in the streets. I'm spending a second straight night at home alone. Curtis was home earlier, but left. The night before he did not come home at all. I heard him talking on the phone, saying he was arrested. He tells the caller there was a car chase. He says he told the police he thought they were robbers and that's why he fled. I do not know what is going on. I do not know why my mother is always in Miami if I'm in Georgia. I do not know why Curtis went to jail the night before. I just know that I am afraid of the strange people I see at the convenience store near the entrance to our complex. I figure they must know I spend nights alone and they are planning to harm me.

When it gets dark, I stay upstairs in the townhouse. I do not know who or what is downstairs anymore. I run some bath water and take a bath. I am nine and lonely and alone here in Atlanta. I jump out of the bathtub, grab a towel, and hustle into my bedroom, where I dry off, turn up the volume on the television set, get under the covers, and fall asleep. I wake up periodically throughout the night. It's always because of the noises. The worst noise is the refrigerator motor. Who knew it could be heard over the din of the blasting television set, over *Hawaii Five-O,* over *Mannix,* over *Ironside?*

In the spring of 1974, my mother and Curtis are home. It's a Saturday but they are still in bed, even though it's almost 11 A.M. I am playing ball with Greg and Anthony, my two new Georgia friends, when they decide to go in the house for some water. I go to their front door, and wait for them to hand me a glass of water. Anthony cracks the door, goes to stick the glass out, but their 150-pound German shepherd comes crashing through the door instead. I take off running. This big brown dog is trying to catch up with me. He's gaining ground and I am running as fast as my little nine-year-old legs and arms can move. I see a dumpster and figure I can get to it and jump inside before the dog catches up with me. I am about fifteen feet from my safe haven, but I know I am meat. He's too close. I reach the dumpster, leap high in the air, and, just as I do, the dog sinks his teeth into my back. It hurts, but not as much as I thought it would.

Greg and Anthony's parents come running out. Their father gets the dog and takes him home. Their mother gets me. We go to my house and try to wake my mother and Curtis. My friends' mother explains what happened, but both are too tired to come to the hospital with me. So Greg and Anthony's mother takes me to the hospital, where the doctors tend to my wounds.

I've had enough of Atlanta. I want something more familiar, like Grandma's bad food in East Cleveland and her crowded house. At least there you do not have to worry about being left alone and vicious dogs.

In a matter of weeks, my wish comes true. For reasons never explained to me, we move back to Cleveland.

◩

Calvin is living in Outhwaite Estate Homes with his mother and Wayne Carter. Antmo is living on Brightwood. I can't live on Brightwood because, for some reason, East Cleveland Schools won't allow me back into Superior Elementary this late in my third-grade year. So instead I am sent to live off St. Clair Avenue in a big, red, three-level apartment building. There are two apartments on each floor. The building is owned by my older cousin Shirley. She is the daughter of Aunt Laura, who died a year earlier. Aunt Laura was smart in business and had acquired several properties, including the building on St. Clair. Shirley lives in one of the units and rents out the other five. On the second floor live Marie and her husband Ron Veasley.

They have an infant girl, whom we all call Buttons. They also now have me to take care of because I will be living here for the remainder of the school year and attending O. W. Holmes Elementary.

I am frightened at the prospect of attending O. W. Holmes. I have heard so many bad things about kids in the big public school system.

Most of the work I can't do because I come to this school with only two months left in the academic year and have missed so much. I pretty much keep to myself, but one day in the coatroom, a boy named Marcus Maddox says he has heard that I want to fight him, which is the last thing I want to do at a new school. Marcus is about my height but stronger.

He takes a swing at me, but somehow I block his punch. He punches again, and again I block it and reflexively hit him with a right cross to the jaw. I punch him five times and everyone sees it. Marcus grabs his coat, cries, and runs off. No one else wants to bother me at O. W. Holmes.

At home, Marie and Ron Veasley are lovey-dovey one moment and fighting the next. Maybe their arguing stems from the fact that they smoke funny cigarettes with Shirley. Shirley appears to sell drugs. Her boyfriend is Homer, a Cleveland police officer. He comes over and smokes marijuana all the time. I think it is so strange that a Cleveland police officer is always smoking dope.

After the school year is over, I move back to Brightwood and am accepted back into Superior Elementary.

I play with my friend Pokey and Antmo, but Dent

mostly hangs around with kids his age from school. Antmo hangs with Dent and the other sixth graders from school sometimes, and with Pokey and me other times.

One day, I am playing with Pokey and I see Marcus Maddox, the boy who picked on me at O. W. Holmes, walking up the street. He says he is moving onto Brightwood. I brag to everybody that I beat him up. I recall for anyone who will listen how he tried to bully me for days and then tried to pick a fight in the coatroom. I describe blow for blow how I blocked his lame punches and countered with some serious blows of my own.

Marcus and I play with his little brother Billy, who is nine, two years our junior. Marcus is growing at a faster pace than I. We enter fourth grade, and I recount my exploits from the fight for all the fourth graders at Superior Elementary School. I tell them how Marcus tried to dog me out at O. W. Holmes. This is my territory, I tell Marcus, who tries to ignore my bragging. He is afraid of me and I want him to pay for any discomfort I might have had at O. W. Holmes.

After school one day, he accidentally trips me.

Whaddaya do that for? I demand.

He apologizes, but I swing and hit him in the face. He is ready to take his punishment because he knows I swing too fast for him to fight back. He is stronger than me, but he is frightened.

Just then, Betty, his mother, walks out on their porch and sees me intimidating her son in the lawn of the next yard.

Marcus, she yells, you get him or I'm gonna get you!

Marcus looks at me and rage engulfs his body. He is standing about five feet from me and squeezes his fists as tight as possible and runs toward me. I know I won't be able to stop him because of his strength.

I'll pulverize you! he screams. I didn't know what that big word meant, but I didn't have time to decipher it anyway.

Next thing I know, Marcus has slammed me to the ground, and then he's on top of me and punching. I'm trying to get loose, but I can't. Antmo and other kids are watching, but they are not about to intervene in a fair, one-on-one fight. Marcus punches me ten, twenty times, and then Betty calls him off.

I skulk home, embarrassed by the beating and by the way I have been treating Marcus. I am mad at myself for not quitting while I was ahead, while I had beaten him and earned his respect. I had to keep picking on him until I got my come-uppance.

Good thing about it is that Marcus is a much more gracious winner than I. Several days later, we make up and are playing again, although the entire neighborhood knows now that I can't beat him. Word even spreads to Superior Elementary School, which really shames me because I have been telling all the girls how I had beaten him.

◫ Four ◫

Calvin's mother and stepfather are getting tired of living in the projects and want to buy a run-down, vacant, two-family home they have seen halfway between East Cleveland and downtown. The three-level, turn-of-the-century house is across the street from the home of Grandma's sister, Aunt Bessie. Pat and Wayne Carter can't afford to buy the house—neither one of them works—so Grandma and Leroy end up purchasing it. They get a loan from First Federal Savings and Loan.

The place is dusty and dirty, but big and elegant. With a little work, it clearly can be a real steal.

Part of that work befalls Antmo, Calvin, and me. We paint, nail loose boards, sweep, mop, cut grass, and move leftover junk to the curb so the rubbish folks can pick it up.

By that fall, it is ready to be inhabited. Grandma rents out one side to an elderly couple named Mr. and Mrs. Johnson. Mrs. Johnson's sister also lives with them. The other half goes to my mother, her new boyfriend Roy Williams, and me.

I am so happy to be living with my mother again, after first being with Marie and then with Grandma since returning from Atlanta in the spring of 1974. My mother is again a unit clerk at St. Vincent Charity Hospital. Roy finds work wherever he can, at a small clothing store on the far East Side of Cleveland, at an after-hours bar as a card dealer, at Pepsi driving a pop truck. I am in the fifth grade, and, for the first time, feeling like part of a real nuclear family. Roy has a daughter, Nikki, about four years younger than me. We get along well when she visits. I am thinking I have a mother now, a stepfather, and a stepsister. I am so happy. But that happiness is short-lived. I start to notice long blue marks on my mother's arms, and I realize she is doing drugs. As a result, she is counting on me to be more independent. She is always telling people that she wants me to be a little man. That's her way of saying I am supposed to be able to help take care of myself. I wash and iron my own clothes at age eleven. I navigate the region of more than two million people with my bus pass.

My mother starts accusing me of doing things I didn't do, stealing things I didn't steal. It happens anytime she needs a fix, anytime she wants some dope and can't get it. Whenever she does get some dope and shoots it, she sits on the little black recliner in our living room and tries to talk to me, but mostly she dozes off. She wakes up suddenly and just picks up conversation where she left off, and gets mad if I can't follow it.

What bothers me is when she is jumpy and picks fights. Fights with her are unfair, of course, because I am just an eleven-year-old kid and she is the adult.

As her drug habits spins out of control, my independence increases as well. She says she is just trying to prepare me for the real world. What I think is that she can't handle the real world and she escapes by shooting heroin.

◻

Antmo and I are visiting Calvin at the public-housing apartment he shares with his mother and stepfather. We have been playing football when we get tired and decide to go back to Calvin's apartment. Antmo heads for the refrigerator for some cold water. I dash up the stairs to the second floor.

Go back downstairs! Wayne Carter screams. I freeze on the stairs and look at Wayne in the bathroom. He has elastic tied around his bicep. And he is sticking a long needle into his vein.

Our eyes lock on one another. I am looking at Wayne shoot the dope into his body. Go back downstairs, he hollers. I want to, but I am frozen, stuck in the same motion of running up the stairs that I had been when I saw him.

Dwayne, get out of here! Wayne hollers again, never once taking the needle out of his arm.

Slowly, I back down the stairs. I do not turn around. Just walk backward, the vision of the needle and the syringe and the tubes and his arm ingesting it all over-whelming me.

I tell Antmo about it, and he suggests we go outside and play so we will not be in the house when Wayne finishes. Wayne has always been nice to me, encouraging me in sports. I had known that he and Pat and my mother shoot dope. I see the marks on their arms and hear their conversations. But this is the first time the whole crazy mess has been so vivid.

Calvin does not know the harm that dope can do. When he and Wayne's nieces see the adults go in the room, they just figure no one is supervising them and they can have unrestricted playtime. Calvin and Ro-Ro, the young daughter of Wayne's older sister, sometimes even tie a belt around their own tiny arms and imitate the adults. Calvin and Ro-Ro call it the needle-in-the-arm thing; it's a game in these Cleveland housing projects. They are punished whenever they get caught playing the game.

◪

I can handle the life of a drug addict's son, but I feel sorry for Calvin. He is younger and doesn't need these hassles. His father obviously feels the same way. Big Calvin lives in Queens now, not far from La Guardia Airport. He has lived in the New York area since shortly after Calvin's birth. He has given up his factory job for the life of a hustler, the underground economy—doing what exactly, I don't know—but he drives a Jaguar and a Rolls Royce and other big fancy cars. He also has a lot of money whenever he returns to Cleveland. Eventually Big Calvin returns to Cleveland and takes custody of Little Calvin, who moves away from me for the first time.

I am sad that my cousin lives out of state, but I know Big Calvin doesn't shoot heroin and will take care of him.

◪

By the spring of 1977, I have found a new source of inspiration and pleasure: organized sports. Along with Michael Singleton, my best friend and classmate, I sign up for the East Cleveland Little League Baseball Program. We both get our permission slips signed and turn them in and show up for the first practice. Mike and I are on the same team and we are assigned to the Reds, a first-year team with a first-year coach, Mr. Maxwell.

We practice several times a week in the early spring, and then we play twice a week once the season starts. Baseball just stretches my days even further. I leave my Superior Avenue home around 7:15 A.M. most mornings, catch my three buses, and try to make it to school by 8:30. I am late a lot. I go to classes all day and then head to Brightwood, where I hang out until it's time for my baseball games. I dress for my game and go to Mike's house, where we both walk to the fields in our Reds outfits. Along the way, people smile and stop us and ask us where we play. I love the attention of being in uniform.

We play our game and, afterward, usually head for an ice cream cone at a stand across from the field. From there, I make a thirty-minute walk to Lakeview and Superior for my bus home. If we play in the late game, I don't arrive home until close to 10 P.M. My mother and Roy criticize my schedule and say they don't know how I get my schoolwork done. My secret is that I am not getting my homework done.

My mother never comes to any of my Little League games. Occasionally, she or Roy will pick me up at

Grandma's house on Brightwood if my team plays the late game. Otherwise, I catch the bus at Lakeview and Superior, even though it's a dangerous area. One night, right where I catch my bus, someone robs the fish store and shoots and kills the owner's daughter. Still, night after night, I walk there in my little Reds uniform and take the bus home.

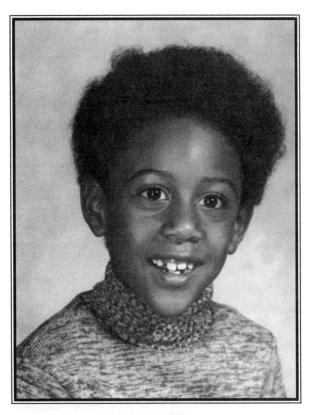

Dwayne, 1970

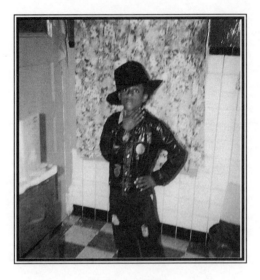

Dwayne, 1969

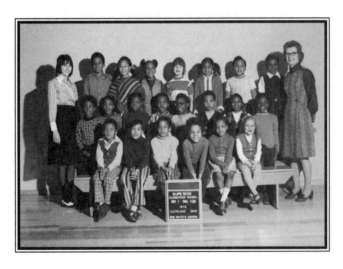

Dwayne's first grade class picture, 1972
Dwayne is in the second row, far left.

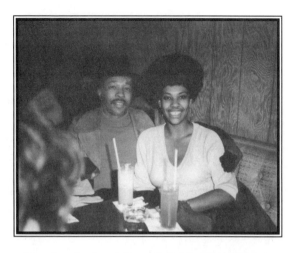

Dwayne's mother, Queenie Bray, with boyfriend Murray Tyson, 1971

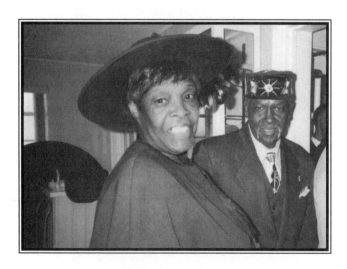

Grandmother Sangenella, 1998

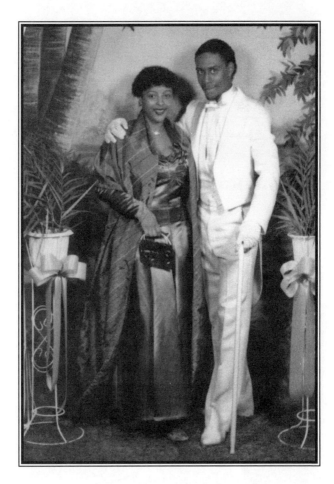

Prom photo of Dwayne and Natalie, June 1983

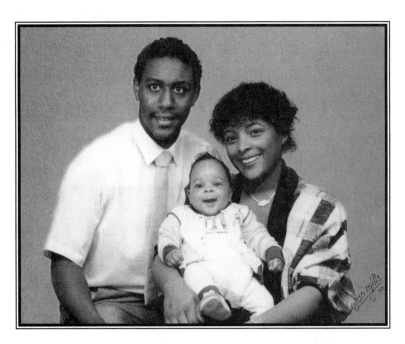

Dwayne, Natalie and Dwayne Jr., 1986

PART

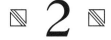 **2**

All the stories I have heard about Kirk Junior High School being large and fast-paced seem true. My body has not grown much since fifth grade and I am clearly still a young boy, even though I am thirteen. Many others at Kirk are men already. They have muscles and deep voices. Some of them even have hair on their faces, under their armpits, and on their chests. I have fourth-grade muscles, a kid's voice, and no signs of peach fuzz.

There are two things I do have: an interest in sports and the stamp of approval for being from the mean streets of Brightwood.

My study habits are extremely poor. Not only have I gotten off to a bad start academically, but it is clear that I am not going to excel in either of the main sports at Kirk: football and basketball. Baseball is my sport, but Kirk does not have a baseball team. Nor does East Cleveland have any summer teams for kids my age, so I will have to wait two years, until the ninth grade, to play organized baseball again. This means there will be little to keep me occupied.

My grades have fallen to mostly Cs and Ds. To my teachers, especially Mr. Capas, the social studies teacher, I am the poster boy for underachievement. Why? Because Mr. Capas has seen me debate points on government policy in his class. He cannot believe I am at the bottom of my unit at Kirk academically.

I am walking down the hall, going to Mr. Duffy's English class, when a girl comes up to me.

Mr. Capas spent a long time in class talking about you, Dwayne. He said you should be in our group, with the smart kids, but that you are lazy and don't want to do the work and that is why you are in such a low group.

I don't even know this girl and try to brush off her comments. But they cling to me like a bad cold. Why would a teacher spend so much time talking about me? It isn't fair for him to go around telling other students I'm a failure.

Earlier that week, students had been assigned to five different groups based on their academic ability. Mr. Capas and several other teachers felt I should have been in the first group, with the smartest kids. But based on my grades and attitude toward doing work, I am placed in the fifth group, the lowest, borderline retarded. I am grouped with kids who don't regularly go to class, who have learning disabilities, and who have been in trouble with the law. Most of these kids can barely read, and I am taking classes with them even though I read at the tenth-grade level two years ago. Being lumped with the dummies makes me even more disinterested in academics. The teachers are sick of it and adopt a no-tolerance policy with my behavior.

One day I am kicked out of science class for disturbing other students who are there actually trying to learn. On my way to the principal's office, I run into three other troublemakers in the hallway. Dorian Hill, David Jones, and Deverick Duncan are plotting something. David says, We're going to pull the fire alarm. You with us?

The alarms sit inside red boxes that hang on the walls. When you pull the lever it leaves bright red paint on your hands and, according to legend, only the fire department can remove it. But Dorian, a light-skinned kid whom I like and so do a number of the girls, says he has some of the special remover. Deverick, fresh out of juvenile prison, is set to do it. So is David Jones.

You in, Bray? one of them asks.

These guys know I'm from Brightwood and that Brightwood kids aren't afraid to have a little fun. I am tempted to join in, but then I realize my convenient excuse. I am wearing a full-length cast on my right leg. The doctor says I have Osgood Slaughter, a bone disease that affects many adolescents and teenagers during growth-spurt years. Wear the cast for six weeks, the doctor says, and the problem will fix itself.

Uh, my leg. I have this damn cast on. I would only slow y'all down, probably get caught.

Yeah, David says. Okay, you go to the office. We'll give you time to get in there.

I hobble down the grand circular staircase of the old building and head to the principal's office. I tell the secretary I have been kicked out of class for making noises and she tells me to have a seat. Just as my bottom lands against the blue porcelain chair, I hear a loud ring.

The principal comes running out of his office, yelling, Everybody out! Everybody out!

The next day, I am called to the principal's office and told that they have caught the three culprits and that I am an accomplice. I deny it and the secretary verifies that I was in the office when the alarm sounded. I am cleared and sent back to class with a warning. All three other guys are expelled.

I go to class every day with kids who can barely read. It is such a waste of time. My worst time is always in Mr. Capas's social studies class. Mr. Capas is almost beet red when I walk through his door. He doesn't want to look at me, he is so disgusted. He gives rudimentary lessons to these kids and they still cannot get the answers right. Every time he asks a question, I raise my hand, but he refuses to acknowledge me for the longest time. Then one day, he tears into me.

Dwayne, you don't even belong in here, he says. You are not allowed to answer questions. When you start to live up to your potential and move into a higher group where you belong, I will allow you to answer questions.

I want to change but . . .

◩

Reverend Smith, the preacher who lives next door to Mama, always tells me, Idle hands are the devil's workshop. He means, of course, that if you don't have anything to do you could end up doing something destructive.

With baseball out of my life, I am a thirteen-year-old who feels his only purpose in life has evaporated. No more getting up in the morning, thinking about that afternoon's baseball game. No more going to school, waiting for the 2:45 P.M. bell so I can go home and change into my baseball uniform. No more showing up at Shaw Field or Patterson Park and taking batting and fielding practice.

So I begin searching trouble out, and my good friend Eric is more than happy to help.

Eric is one of the unreachable kids on the lowest academic rung. He's not dumb but thinks he's too cool, too smooth to pay attention and learn. That's for chumps, not for Eric; and, I guess I've decided it's not for me. I hang out with Eric because he's popular with some of the more adventurous girls and he dresses nicely. I do not dress sharply anymore because my mother doesn't buy me nice clothes like she once did. She is addicted to heroin and that has altered our relationship. When I was young, I was her trophy child. She doted on me, flaunting the fact that I had soft curly hair and eyelashes longer than most women in mascara. But now I am a thirteen-year-old, not the precocious little boy all of East Cleveland seemed to fuss over. And she is a twenty-seven-year-old junkie.

Eric and I plan to meet at his house after school.

Hey, dog, you know I got three buses to catch to get home, I tell him.

Stay on Brightwood overnight, he urges.

I can't do that. I don't have no clothes over there.

Just come over to my crib after school with me.

I do as he suggests, going to his house on Roxbury Avenue, which is two streets over from Brightwood. We get there and Eric shows me his brother's stash of marijuana. Wanna get high? he asks.

That's your brother's shit, I say.

He don't care. He sells this shit. He got a lot of it. We can roll up a joint.

He leaves the room and comes back with a little brown package that has E-Z Wider written over it. He pulls out a sheet of paper, opens it, and sprinkles the green-brown grass in it. He rolls it up, and I am impressed. I have seen Bill and Bobby and Antmo do this but I have never tried it. After Eric rolls up the joint, he puts the whole thing in his mouth and licks it. I do not know why, but I have seen Bill and Bobby do that, too.

Eric is thirteen like me. He is wearing Stacey Adams shoes and a cashmere button-down sweater. He has on Pierre Cardin fragrance and is talking about all his alleged sexual conquests. I'm still a virgin.

Eric lights the joint, raises it to his lips, takes a deep drag, chokes a little—like Bill and Bobby—and hands the joint to me.

This some good shit, he says.

I have never had a joint in my hands. Bill, Bobby, and Antmo let me drink but not smoke.

I don't want Eric to know that I have never smoked reefer. He is still choking from his drag. He coughs, bends over slightly, and swivels around.

Whoa! he says.

Now he admonishes me. Smoke that shit before it burns up.

I put the joint to my lips, breathe in and cough, but never inhale because I don't know how. I just breathe in, hold the smoke and blow it out, never inhaling.

Eric does not seem to notice and we finish the joint and I get up to leave, reeking of pot.

One good thing about living on Superior with my mother and Roy is that they rented out the back room of our duplex to Prince, my mother's first cousin. It's the mid-1970s, and Prince is part of the in-crowd on the East Side of Cleveland. His bedroom, which essentially is all he gets for his fifty dollars-a-month rent, is on the second floor, directly behind mine. You have to go through my bedroom to get to his. Prince's room is adorned with all kinds of lights, including fluorescent. He has mirrors hanging on the wall. I am impressed and Prince is, to me, the slickest cat in the world. While I never associate with any of the kids my age in this neighborhood, Prince grew up here. He has a lot of friends here—make that girlfriends.

Prince is two years younger than my mother. He loves to talk about his sexual conquests with anybody, which includes me. He tells me of the many times he has sex with women and brags constantly about his social life. And now that his bedroom is next to mine, he tells me that I would get to see all of his women firsthand, as they come to his pleasure den. Do I ever. Prince doesn't have as many women as his boasting would suggest—it's not like there is a different lady tromping through my bedroom on a nightly basis to get to his lair. But at least once a week, a new woman sashays into our front door, speaks softly, and heads up the stairs to socialize with my cousin. These dates of Prince's are usually in their early or late twenties, like Prince. Even if I'm not sleepy, I know it's time to go to bed. Prince plays soft music and burns incense. The smell of burning marijuana wafts under the door into my room and surrounds me as I lie in my full-sized bed. I hear giggling and the lights go out. Then there's grunting and the sound of pressure being put on the slats of Prince's bed.

When Prince isn't working as a nurse at the downtown Cuyahoga County Jail and when he isn't luring women to his room, he coaches a summer league basketball team. One player on the team is James Calvin Wilson. J. C. is on scholarship at the University of Pittsburgh, where he rooms with Tony Dorsett, one of the nation's top college running backs and a candidate for the Heisman Trophy. I love being around these jocks, watching them play basketball and then gather at my house afterward to socialize with Prince and the women.

I am the team manager, which means after each

game I walk around the locker room and pick up all the players' sweaty jerseys, shorts, and jockstraps. Every now and then, several members of the Cleveland Cavaliers will show up and play on one of the opposing teams. The Cavs players are just staying in shape during the off-season, and the basketball here isn't bad at all. The games are played at a recreational center in the heart of Cleveland's East Side. During the action, Prince paces the sidelines and jaws with the referee like this is the NBA. He has a clipboard and shuffles his players in and out of the games. Crowds of about a hundred folks are on hand. I find it strange that many folks root against Bobby Bingo Smith and some of the other Cavs. I have never seen anyone in Cleveland root against the Cavs, except Leroy, Grandma's husband. But I think even he likes them. He just roots for the other team during NBA games because he thinks all Cleveland sports teams are destined to disappoint their fans.

By July, J. C. has to leave and return to college. Several times over the next few months, however, Pitt plays on national TV and I watch J. C. cover receivers. That is the case one October Saturday when Leroy and I are watching the game.

That interception was by James Calvin Wilson, the nifty little cornerback out of East Tech High School in Cleveland, Ohio, ABC's Keith Jackson says with a twang. I am jumping around the living room yelling, I know him! I know him! He's been over to my house! Walked through my bedroom! Gave me his autograph! I spent the summer with him!

You don't know him, Bray, Leroy says.

Uh, huh! I'm telling you, we're just like cousins.

Leroy laughs and calls Grandma. Bray know this man here on the television, he tells his wife.

Ain't that sweet, Grandma says.

Over the next few months I follow J. C.'s career through the sports pages and the TV. He makes several college all-star teams and is drafted in the fifth round by the Houston Oilers. He quickly becomes a starting player and I root for him even more, except for twice a year. That's when the Oilers play the Cleveland Browns, an opponent in their division.

I like living at 7209 Superior, even after Prince and my mother decide it's time for him to move out. Our big beige-and-brown wood house is spacious and clean inside. Outside, I don't go in the backyard alone much because some very big rats, the size of cats, have claimed that territory. I am forced to take out the garbage back there twice a week and I always do so with a large stick in my hand, in case one of the rodents decides to attack. They never do and appear more afraid of me than I am of them. But I don't want to take any chances. Fortunately, we don't have any rats or mice in our home.

Antmo sleeps over a lot, or I'll sleep over with him on Brightwood. A lot of Roy's friends come over. Most of these men are sports-minded and they seem to like me a lot because I am always watching games on TV.

◻

One Sunday during the summer of 1977, Little Calvin is visiting, along with his mother, Pat, and our mother's close friend Loretta Woods. Our mothers have been doing a lot of whispering and huddling all morning and then they make what they call "a run." I know that means they want to score some drugs, but Calvin is ten and I am not sure he really understands.

Calvin and I are watching TV when our parents and

Loretta return. Up the stairs and into the bathroom the women go. They stay up there for a while, maybe more than forty-five minutes. Loretta comes back downstairs with us. We are sitting on our sofa, facing the television. Loretta is trying to hold a conversation but she seems drowsy and keeps dozing off.

My mother comes downstairs, too, and she seems more alert. She peeks in on us and goes to start dinner. Suddenly, Loretta loses consciousness and falls in Calvin's ten-year-old lap. Calvin is frightened.

What's wrong with her? What's wrong with her? Calvin wants to know

I call my mother and at the same time inch closer to Loretta. I notice how her lips and extremities appear to be purple, as if all the blood from her body is trying to escape. Her long, black wooly hair is a mess and she is just lying on the couch, flopped down. I reach out and touch her ebony skin. It is warm and soft and smooth. Her brown eyes stand open even though she is unconscious. Her blouse is open, too, and I can see her right breast. I can also see the track marks running the length of her arms.

Her head rests on its right side and saliva pours involuntarily out of a corner of her mouth. Some of the spit falls on the floor while some just rolls down her jaw to her neck and down her body. Her neck appears to be broken.

I have never seen anyone die before my eyes, but I know that is Loretta's fate. I am overwhelmed. Suddenly, my mother and Pat come racing in with ice cubes in their hands. They are rubbing the ice over Loretta's body.

C'mon, Loretta, girl, wake up! my mother says.

Pat's urging her, too.

Loretta! Loretta! Loretta!

C'mon, girl, Pat says.

Loretta!

Calvin fades to the background, stunned, a ten-year-old boy growing harder every second.

Loretta!

Finally, I say, I'm gonna get some help!

I get up and run toward our front door. Outside, I have two options as I stare at the mid-afternoon traffic passing along busy Superior Avenue. Both are on the other side of the street.

I could run over to Aunt Bessie's house. She lives almost directly across from us, but she knows my mother and Roy do drugs and I doubt that she wants to get involved with one of their overdosing friends. Two properties to the left of Aunt Bessie's house is Fire Station No. 20. Not only are engines and ladders there, but paramedics as well.

The doors to the firehouse are locked, and why wouldn't they be? This is Seventy-second Street and Superior, one of the meanest neighborhoods in a mean city. I bang on the door. A white man with white hair in blue pants and a blue shirt finally opens the door.

Help! Help! I scream. She ain't breathing. I need help!

I have run over to the fire station in about fifteen seconds. You would think they would grab their bags and run back over to our house.

They don't.

Instead, they raise the firehouse door, sound an alarm, and prep for an emergency. A fire engine and ambulance, both loaded with firefighters, pull out of the station for the thirty-five-yard dash to my front door.

They are dressed in full firefighter gear: the heavy yellow raincoats, the red helmets, the black boots. The medics bring in their bags and I feel lucky they do not use the axes on our wooden screen door. They take Loretta's pulse and, as far as I can tell, she does not

DWAYNE BRAY

have one. They cup her mouth and nose with an oxygen mask, slide a board underneath her, wrap a white sheet around her, and haul her out of the house. By the time they reach the porch, Loretta comes to. She is disoriented and fights with the medics.

Y'all get the hell off me, she says.

She fights and fights and finally they give up. Right there on the porch, she gets up and off the stretcher. She refuses any further medical assistance. My mother tells the medics that whatever it is that turned on Loretta like that, she had taken it before she got to our home. They leave, without calling the police.

After the firefighters leave, my mother calls me into her room.

You don't ever bring the PO-lice into my house. Ever. Do you hear me, boy?

After she scolds me, she finishes dinner, feeds me, and she and Pat huddle.

I gotta go get me and you some that dope, girl, she tells her younger sister.

To the heroin addict, whenever they see someone overdose, they want some. That's good dope, to them. They just know not to take as much.

�△

Not all of our crises involve drugs. One day Roy is driving south on Warrensville Center Road, heading toward suburban Shaker Heights. Without explanation, a car pulls up beside us and the driver—a young, white male—leans toward the passenger side and hollers through the rolled-down window.

Nigger!

A young white woman is in the passenger seat and

perhaps some other people in the back seat. After the driver delivers his expletive, he races down the road.

I am stunned, and so is my mother. Roy accelerates the big, gray Electra 225 and gives chase.

Let him go, Roy, my mother urges. Roy doesn't say much, just drives until, several blocks up the road, he sees the harasser's car stopped at a traffic light behind several other cars.

Roy positions our car next to his. Reaching under the seat, Roy says, Give me the gun, Queenie! Give me the gun!

My mother is saying, No, Roy, don't shoot him.

Roy is reaching under the seat, scrambling for something. I'm aware that the only thing under the seat is a steering-wheel locking device, not a gun. The driver of the other car doesn't know that. He starts apologizing. His front-seat female companion starts pleading with Roy.

Mister, don't shoot us, he didn't mean it. Please, mister, he doesn't know what he's saying. Don't shoot.

Give me the gun, Queenie! Roy demands, feigning looking for a pistol. My mother is playing the role, too, pleading with Roy not to shoot the young racist.

After Roy has humiliated the man enough, Roy just pulls off. Funny thing is, no one in our car laughs or gets a kick out of frightening the young man.

N

I never go to the ninth grade, not for a full year anyway. Shortly after school starts in September 1979, East Cleveland teachers go on strike. I don't sweat the work stoppage—I'm glad to have a longer summer vacation.

No one is living at our house on Superior. Roy has moved. He and my mother had begun arguing all the time over unpaid bills and other problems. I'm upset with my mother for allowing our family to split. I start spending the night on Brightwood and she reconciles with Roy at his new apartment. I go back home one day and stay the night alone. Somehow, mice have made their way into our house. I pack a suitcase and head to Grandma's house for good.

About a week later, I'm watching TV when Grandma's first husband, my maternal grandfather, calls from Meridian, Mississippi. He has been keeping tabs on me over the years, and knows things aren't going too well here, so I agree to move to Meridian with him. He says I can go to school during the week and work with him on his construction crew on Saturdays. Becoming a laborer for the bricklayers sounds like an attractive offer.

◩

My grandfather, whom I call Daddy, lives in a house located across from a substation power plant. He lives in the city, but most of the surrounding property, much of which he owns, is made up of shacks. Daddy's house is larger than the others, with three bedrooms and bricked in a crude fashion. Daddy bricked it himself, but he didn't spend time on it like he does with those houses he gets paid to brick.

Daddy and Dot, his wife, sleep in one room. Their daughter Ferleisi, my aunt, is a tenth grader, and she sleeps in another room. And I get the large front room with the king-size bed. I have a black-and-white portable television, which I watch until the *Tonight Show with Johnny Carson* is over.

When Daddy gives me my blue transcript paper from Shaw High School, it says grade ten. He tells me to just forget about ninth grade because in Mississippi they allow you to go to your true grade. East Cleveland had made me start kindergarten a year late, so Daddy says he is "undoing this injustice." I'm on his soil, in the South, and he can pull strings for me. I know better, though. I know I'm not supposed to be in the tenth grade. But I keep my mouth shut and go along with the plan.

At first, I have some adjusting to do at Harris Campus, which is the school for tenth graders. It is part of Meridian High School, but only the juniors and seniors attend classes on the main campus. I often wake up late and frequently miss the 7:30 A.M. school bus that carries us over the hilly Meridian landscape to Harris Campus. When I wake up early enough to make the bus, I have to listen to a large fifteen-year-old country boy named Frankie, who sits in the back with a lot of other wide-awake Southern teenagers.

Cle-e-e-velan! he shouts every time I get on board. Boy, tell me, hah dose ol' Cl-e-e-velan Browns gone do?

Frankie and several other boys are pretty cool. Not like the dudes I know back in Cleveland, but they aren't bad for a bunch of country kids. And they are all thick, while I'm still skinny, maybe 135 pounds.

I'm not part of the best and brightest at Harris Campus, but I manage to pass most of my classes with Cs and some Ds. I start off getting Fs in algebra. This is because at Shaw in East Cleveland I was still a year away from algebra, but now that I have skipped a grade, I have to take it.

Another student and I start making bets on our daily algebra quiz. Who's going to get the highest score? We bet mostly just milk money, but the competition brings out the best in me and pretty soon I'm scoring in the high 80s. Next thing you know my daily quiz scores in algebra are in the 90s, As. I haven't made As in anything since fourth grade. But competition pushes me to excel. This is where I first learn the value of good, friendly competition. If you have something to shoot for, someone to beat, you do better.

In addition to going to work with Daddy, I spend a lot of my time playing tennis with a boy named Daryl from around the corner. Daryl, like me, is from the North. His mother lives in Chicago, but she sent him to Meridian to live with his maternal grandparents so he could escape the gang life of the Windy City. Like me, Daryl is skinny, but he is more gangly. We're both athletic and start playing almost daily matches of tennis. We walk a half mile up sloping hills to Meridian High School and hit on the little green ball. Several times we play four sets an afternoon. We both become pretty good at the game.

Daryl talks about trying out for the tennis team, but I want none of it. My love is baseball and I wait for baseball tryouts. Meridian has a great baseball tradition, and at least a dozen guys in the major leagues and the minor leagues are former members of the Meridian Wildcats. I know I've had a long layoff from baseball—two years—and I'm rusty. I go out for the team but get cut after three weeks of intense practice. I am devastated.

◫

I like working with Daddy but it's hard. We get up early and head to the construction site by 7:30 A.M. That way, we can get a couple of hours under our belts before the sun starts blazing. Of all the guys on the crew, I like Buddy the most. Buddy is a dark-skinned man in his mid-twenties. He has served time in prison and Daddy hired him when he was released. Daddy feels he's doing a community service when he hires ex-cons. He puts these men to work so they won't have to go back to their old ways. Many straighten themselves out; others don't.

I'm not sure why Buddy had been locked up at Parchman, the infamous prison in Mississippi, but he is now Daddy's right-hand man.

Daddy is the licensed, independent contractor. He has taught most of the crew of about a dozen how to perform the bricklaying work. My job is to fill the wheelbarrow with bricks and deliver them to each side of whatever structure we are enclosing. Sometimes it's an office building, but mostly it's a new house in the countryside.

I am afraid of heights. One day, I load the wheelbarrow and both the wheelbarrow and I are loaded onto the scaffold and lifted to about the fourth story of the building. The scaffolding seems to have been put up too quickly, at least for my tastes, and is shaking. I'm frightened.

Look at Little Bray, one of the men calls out.

Damn, says another. He's shaking more than the scaffold.

Everybody laughs, but when I am sent down for another load of bricks I refuse to go back up. I settle on another task.

◪

What I find most remarkable about Daddy is how he communicates with people. He seems to have a good rapport with the poor black laborers who work for him, but he also speaks the language of the wealthy white home-buyers and developers.

One day, we have driven out to an all-white section of Meridian in Daddy's white-and-yellow Ford pickup truck, which has to be a decade old. There is Daddy in his work boots and workman pants and shirt. He is talking to a very tanned white man who is dressed in loafers, a golf shirt, and expensive slacks. The man has on a gold watch and ring. He reeks of money.

I couldn't understand how that had happened, Sammy, the man says to Daddy.

Yeah, Daddy says, that perplexed me too.

Per-*what*? I thought. What's that word he's using? I rush into the house when we get home and find a dictionary.

It says: per-plex v. To confuse; bewilder.

From that point on, I listen to Daddy as he talks to business people, both black and white. I begin to understand the power of language but I don't understand where he has picked up all these words.

◫

By the first part of 1980, my official transcript finally shows up in the principal's office. I'm called to explain the grade discrepancy. A group of four administrators is standing around when I get to the office. They close the door and ask me if I know that I'm supposed to be in the ninth grade, not tenth. I 'fess up.

This is the biggest scam ever pulled on Meridian Schools, claims the principal.

I'm just waiting to see what the damage is going to be. But the principal surprises me. He looks at my grades, and says that because I'm passing all my tenth-grade classes—just barely, but passing—he's going to leave me in the tenth grade.

If you want to graduate with the tenth graders in two years, you betta work yo tail off, son, he says.

Yes, sir, I say. It's the first time I remember addressing any authority figure as sir. All the country kids always answer adults, Yes, sir, or Yes, ma'am. But I'm from Cleveland and when an adult calls on me I just say, Huh?

By March, Daddy and I aren't getting along. I love Daddy and respect his work ethic. He has made a lot from nothing: never finishing high school, going straight into the service during the Korean War, coming home and learning to lay bricks. But he can also be moody, especially after he gets a few drinks in him. He wants to be a disciplinarian, something I thought I needed. But I have been on my own too long in Cleveland to start taking orders from a father figure at this point in my life. At least that's how I feel. He has reduced my allowance from ten dollars a week to nothing at all most weeks. He doesn't take me to work with him any longer and I am broke and lonely. The honeymoon is over. Mississippi makes me feel like I'm in prison for no other reason than I'm homesick.

I call my mother. She sends bus fare because Daddy doesn't want me to go and I'm afraid to ask him for it. When school ends in May, I buy a ticket and prepare to go back to Cleveland.

Daddy just lies on the couch, tears in his eyes. He thought I had come to live with him forever. But I can't. I don't like it here in Mississippi.

Bye, Daddy, I say, planting a big kiss on his cheek above the stream of tears rolling down his face.

Bye, son, he says.

I'm going home, just like when I left Atlanta. Only this time, I have watched Daddy in action and I think I now know what manhood is about. At least I've formed goals. I want to get an education, a house some day, and be somebody. Just like Daddy. He has taught me a lot.

◪

Home on Brightwood never looked so beautiful. The
Greyhound bus trip back to Cleveland lasts about twenty-
two hours. When I get off the bus, cousin Prince comes
downtown to pick me up. Antmo and Unc are the only
two at home when I get there. Grandma is at church. It's
the first Sunday in June 1980.

By that following winter, I am plodding along academically as usual. For all I've learned from Daddy, I still
haven't figured out how to improve my study habits.
When time for spring sports tryouts comes, I have to
choose between baseball and tennis. I played so much
tennis in Meridian with Daryl that I am doubtless one of
the top players at an innercity school like Shaw High. But
I again choose baseball over tennis and we begin practice
in February. At least here in East Cleveland I'm a known
commodity. This is where I played Little League and
made the all-star teams. I am placed on the junior varsity
and after one game moved up to the varsity, where I
become a starter for the season. It's not a good season as
we lose all but two of our two dozen games. But I'm only
in the tenth grade and realize I have two more years of
high school baseball to go. I am happy I came back home.

◪

Ivan rarely wears a shirt in the hot Cleveland weather,
and his wide belly hangs over his beltless, cut-off jeans.
He lives on Penrose Avenue, the street immediately west
of Brightwood. For years I have faced Ivan in the regular
Brightwood-Penrose games of tackle football, but now the
game is craps.

Ivan, all 230-odd pounds of him, is kneeling over the

dice. I have him faded for a ten-dollar shot.

C'mon, seven, light 'em up, Ivan says. He laughs deviously, his confidence readily apparent. The scruffy white dice are chipped on the corners, and this seems to assure Ivan that he can throw any point he wants. He's looking for a seven or eleven, first-roll winners. The bones roll off his right fingertips and across the block. One bumps off my shoe. It should be a one. The other dice shows a two.

Craps, I say.

Bullshit, Ivan snaps. You caught 'em. You stuck yo foot out, Bray.

He laughs, as if he has gotten the better of me. He is at least eighty pounds heavier than I am and much stronger. He knows I can argue with him but that is about all I can do.

I reach down for the twenty dollars, my ten and his ten. Man, you rolled those dice into my feet, and they are part of the game.

Don't touch my fuckin' money, he says menacingly.

C'mon, Ivan, don't be pulling that bullshit, I say. You know you crapped out.

Ivan repeats himself. Don't touch my fuckin' money, Bray.

Now I'm stuck. If I let him get away with this, I'll be chumped in front of all the other crap players, who might next want to take me on. If I challenge him, I run the risk of him slamming me into the concrete. People around here don't play about money, especially not Ivan.

Ivan gives me an out. He asks Dan, my friend, who's right.

I ain't in this mess.

I'm thinking, Thanks a lot, Dan. Don't forget you came here with me.

In street dice, it's better to keep your mouth shut if

you're not part of the dispute.

Shoot the shit over, I finally say to Ivan.

Ivan laughs. He gets low to the ground and shakes the dice. I'm staring at the top of his head, which is full of nappy hair. He rolls the dice. One lands with a single dot face up and the other lands on a two.

Craps again, I say. I scoop up his ten and mine.

Bet back, he says quickly, irritated.

Bet back, big boy, I challenge him.

He rolls the dice out once more and they go outside the block. Out of play. He has to try again. Twelve.

Craps again, I call out, exalting in his spate of bad luck, scooping up his ten once more.

Ivan rears back, slams the dice against the side of the old green-and-white house, and announces he's done. This is good for me, because Ivan always seems to get the best of me at this game. I can beat the others but it's Ivan and his bullying tactics—i.e., cheating—that always has me on the ropes.

Four or five other guys are in the game. Dan and I are both winning and trying not to bet against one another. We have been at it for about five or six hours now, too long for me to keep track. It is closing in on midnight, and I'm on Penrose. Our two streets no longer feud.

Rollers! someone shouts.

This craps game is in the driveway on the side of a vacant house. When the lookout spots the police rolling slowly down Penrose, we all carefully walk to the back of the house. This scene, with the cops rolling down on us, plays itself out two or three times during any game that lasts this long. East Cleveland police pull slowly in front of the house and shine a bright light on the spot where the craps game had been going full-throttle just thirty seconds earlier. We are out of view in the back.

If the cops start to exit their car, we all know to run like hell. I would jump the fence and practically be in my own backyard on Brightwood. Dan would follow me and maybe a few of the others. Some would go their own way. But East Cleveland police would rather see us shooting dice, staying out of any real trouble, and mostly they drive up to let us know they know we're here gambling. I can hear the engine of the car. Everybody with me is quiet, except for the sound of beer and wine going down guys' throats. My heart is thumping and I'm sweating. E.C.P.D pulls off.

I started this game with maybe twenty dollars. We are shooting for five dollars a hand. Dan started with about as much as me. More than a dozen guys have come and gone, like Ivan, and the four remaining are low on cash. Dan and I are winning and each of us has more than one hundred dollars. I have about two hundred dollars, but I don't know that yet because I believe in that Kenny Rogers character: Never count your winnings until the dealin' is done.

I grab a Mickey's malt liquor, pull off the tab, and down about half of it.

Fuck this, I say. Everyone is listening to me because I got all the money. I ain't shootin' no more damn fives. That's chump change. Tens and up.

Boris, a guy from Forest Hills, complains. He doesn't have enough money to cover me for ten dollars a shot. I know that, but I am tired of shooting. I am tired of worrying about the police. I want to get me some food, a cold six-pack, and head back to Brightwood.

No one will fade me and as soon as the game appears over, Dan says, Come on, Bray, I got you.

I glare at him. My look is saying to Dan, *Stupid ass, we came here together. Don't fade me.*

Every man's for himself, says Dan, a dark skinny guy who is one of the best basketball players in the neighborhood. He is two years my senior, but the two of us have become tight. I also know he is slick with the dice and can get hot and take my money quick.

Ten dollars are on the table from both of us. I lock the dice together and roll. Six.

Six-eight, Dan says.

No bet, I say.

My next roll is a six and I win. No one else wants to fade me so I call an end to the game. All the losers walk away and when they do, I pull out my wad of cash. I have $230. Not a bad day's work for an unemployed teenager. Dan has more than a hundred dollars.

Out of nowhere, someone says, Hey, one of y'all got a light?

The voice is coming from the other side of Penrose, about fifteen yards away. A man in his late twenties, someone I have never seen before, is standing almost in front of Ivan's house. He starts walking toward us, mumbling something about a light. I don't smoke and say, Nah, brother.

Dan has a cigarette in his hand. The man keeps coming our way and as he's halfway across the street, Dan hollers, He's got a gun!

Dan and I haul ass and the man with the pistol starts running after us. He apparently doesn't realize we are so close to home. Dan and I run in back of the house where we have been shooting craps, with the stranger about thirty yards off our trail. I am running and nearly trip. Dan leaps over an old wooden fence and lands in Reverend Smith's backyard, next to Grandma's house.

I follow, but this is even worse. Reverend Smith had already told all of us that if he catches us in his backyard with his antique cars and kennel of dogs, he is going to put a plug in our butts with his shotgun. Reverend Smith is a man of the cloth, but he is also a card-carrying member of the National Rifle Association, and he believes strongly in the right to bear arms and use them to protect his property.

It is either be shot by the stick-up man or be shot by Reverend Smith, once my preacher.

I take my chances on Reverend Smith, whom I know. We are in his backyard. It is dark, around 1:30 A.M., and I am stepping in dog feces. His dogs, in a big cage he has built, are barking and going crazy as Dan and I run through the yard. Am I going to get shot from the back by the stranger or from the front by the good reverend? I fall and my arm is now caked in feces. The stick-up man is standing on the other side of the fence, apparently trying to decide if it's worth it to come after us. He has figured out we are in our own territory and know where we're headed.

Finally I jump the fence from Reverend Smith's yard into my own yard. I hide on the side of the house next to Dan and I can hear the reverend in his yard. I'm sure he's armed, but I'm in a safe haven now. I walk to the side of Grandma's house, hop the banister, and sit on the porch. I have $230 in my pocket and dog crap on my arm. This is a tough way to earn money.

�****◆

Most of my friends have steady girlfriends. Antmo is dating Denise McClendon, a girl whose family lives across from ours on Brightwood. Denise has a stepsister, Toya, whom I flirt with all the time. She is kind of fast, which I like. She has pretty brown skin and a well-developed physique for her age. She attracts the attention of older boys. I am finding sixteen to be a tough age. I am supposed to be into girls but most sixteen-year-old girls are into boys eighteen and older. Maybe it's that older boys—men, really—have money and cars and stronger bodies. It seems I was more popular with girls when I was twelve and thirteen than I am now.

Toya, however, is nice to me. We talk at night on the porch and she says she likes me and I think I like her. Their house is a three-level brick structure, one of the finest homes on Brightwood. Undoubtedly it was built in the early 1900s by some wealthy family, one of the city's pioneering clans. That history is lost on Toya and me as we gaze at the stars and fight off the mosquitoes. A couple of times I hold her hand and reveal some of my most intimate thoughts. But I never touch her in a romantic way. I never try to kiss her, or hold her body in my arms, or feel her budding breasts. Eventually, Toya and Denise and the rest of the family move. Denise and Antmo continue their relationship. Denise is my age, too, and the fact that she is dating my eighteen-year-old uncle confirms my point: I am sixteen and can't find a girl to date because all the more experienced boys have them all.

◩

When eleventh grade begins in the fall of 1981, I sit toward the back of my homeroom class. Two rows in front of me is a girl I have never seen before. She has a nice figure and her skin is light brown and the smoothest I have ever seen. This girl whose name I don't know catches me staring at her and smiles. Her teeth are perfectly straight and very white.

The teacher calls the roll. Her name is Natalie Williams.

Over the next week, I pass Natalie in class several times and always say hi. For the first time in years, going to school is fun.

My friend Phyllis comes up to me one day after class. You know Natalie, she says. She wants your phone number. I want to give Phyllis a big hug, but I play it cool.

Our first date takes place at Natalie's house, a small, cluttered suite she shares with her mother and brother. Her mother eventually retires to her bedroom, leaving her daughter with me on the living room couch. We are watching the Oklahoma-Nebraska game. I can't believe I am sitting here with this pretty high school junior. She could have been with an older boy who had a car, but instead she picked me. On top of that, she knows something about sports. I put my arm around her, pull her closer, and we kiss. When we stop fifteen minutes later, the game is over and I have no idea who won. I don't care. I've got a girlfriend.

◨

During the winter of 1982, Grandma buys me a 1971 Chevrolet Impala. The car, dark green and in great shape, belonged to the elderly man who lived on the second floor of Grandma's sister's house. When the man died, Grandma asked his widow if she would sell her the car so I would have something to drive to school. The widow and Grandma have no idea my grades are so God-awful. They only know that it seems like I go to school and never cause anyone any problems. She agrees to sell the car, worth at least a thousand dollars, to Grandma for only one hundred.

I love the Chevy and wash and wax it constantly. I buy Armor-All and spray it on the tires so they gleam. The car is also a way for me to make money. There are a lot of people with a lot of schemes for making money or getting drugs. Usually all they need is a ride and now I have one. After school or on weekends, I am usually working at Dwayne's Taxi Service. Pat, my aunt, is one of my favorite customers. She is now living back in the house on Brightwood, her marriage to Wayne Carter long broken off. She is a regular heroin user and still buys her drugs down in the Cuyahoga Metropolitan Housing Authority projects. That's a long way from Brightwood, and she pays me five to ten dollars a trip every time I give her a lift. This is dangerous work because I sometimes have to sit in a dark housing project parking lot while she runs in to buy her drugs. Sometimes her friends are in the car with me, sometimes Natalie—my new girlfriend—is in the car with me. I feel bad that I have introduced Natalie to this world where people pay you to take them to buy two hundred dollars' worth of dope. But it's a way to keep a few dollars in my pocket.

Another person who uses my taxi service is John, one of my closest friends. John is a few years older than I am. He has already been in and out of jail but we get along famously because we both like to shoot dice.

John also likes to steal meat from grocery stores. So I give him a lift, he goes in and steals his meat, and the two of us go and sell it. I guess I am just as guilty as John for stealing this meat, but I look at it as a way of providing a service. I have a girlfriend and a car, and I need money to keep both of them going.

John steals mostly from Pick & Pay supermarkets in East Cleveland and Cleveland Heights. We nickname the store Pick & Walk because John never actually pays.

One day, John hits a grocery store without me. He gets busted and has to appear before East Cleveland Judge Fred

M. Mosely, who has gained a reputation as a hard-nosed, law-and-order jurist who wants to take the city back from John, Bill, me, and the other criminals and gamblers. Mosely is a southern-born ordained minister and former prosecuting attorney in the antitrust division of the U.S. Department of Justice.

Mosely keeps John in the small, filthy East Cleveland Jail several weeks, even though state law says a prisoner can't be kept in a city jail longer than seventy-two hours. Mosley's Law differs from state law.

It is only a matter of time before Mosely and I meet face-to-face. I am too out of control to stay away from his courtroom for long. I gamble, drive people to dope houses, take them to steal meat, and hang out on corners and drink. Natalie has had some influence on helping me get my life in order, but bad habits are hard to break.

I appear in Mosely's courtroom in the winter of 1982. My court date stems from an accident I had with a big buckeye tree halfway up Brightwood. I had been driving south when the front tires of the Chevy hit a patch of ice. Traffic was coming the opposite direction and I was losing control, so I steered toward the tree to avoid injuring someone in the other cars. Natalie was in the passenger's seat, and her head smashed into the windshield. She was unconscious and paramedics rushed her to Huron Road Hospital. She ended up with a bad headache but other than that was fine. The cops cited me for failure to control my vehicle and reckless operation. The Chevy was wasted.

Judge Mosely doesn't like teenage drivers. After allowing me only a brief explanation of the road conditions, Mosely fines me $140. I feel lucky because several people before me have been fined hundreds of dollars more for seemingly innocuous incidents. Some have even been taken off to jail for minor misdemeanors. Mosely tells me that he knows I probably can't pay the fine. He places me in his penalty-option program, under which I can work off my fine by cleaning up vacant lots or other rundown parts of the city. The administrator gives me a job in the East Cleveland Clerk of Courts office filing papers and giving defendants receipts when they pay off their fines. Some former street acquaintances roll their eyes when they see me behind the big counter. They think I have gone to work for the police.

I am quick to say, I'm just working off a fine, man.

This way, I won't get labeled as a snitch. Still, some of the guys from the streets ask me why they have to shovel snow and clean up the parks to work off their debt to the city, while I get a cushy job inside a warm office.

The late winter of 1982 means the start of another baseball season at Shaw. This is my junior year and I am slated to be the starting center fielder. With three of us juniors returning as starters and a host of other sophomores, juniors, and seniors joining our ranks, we're expected to be much improved over the 1981 season. We start the season off with indoor practices in Shaw's Korb Gymnasium every Sunday morning. It is March 7, our second Sunday of practice. We take fielding practice, turning double plays on the basketball court. The ball bounces high and hard off the hardwood, but I like it because it reminds me of practice with the country boys in Meridian. There is also a batting cage with a machine hurling 75 m.p.h. fastballs our way. During a break, I overhear a couple of the other players chatting. They are looking downcast, not their normally rowdy selves.

Why is everyone so quiet? I ask.

Haven't you heard? someone says. Reggie Brooks is dead. His father shot him and his two brothers last night while they were sleeping.

I had met Reggie a couple times, first back when we were about twelve and both trying out for the East Cleveland Chiefs football team. Reggie was strong and quick. He played running back and would mow me down when I came up from my cornerback position and tried to tackle him. I had also played basketball against him in a league at the East Cleveland YMCA.

Many of my baseball teammates also are on the football team, as was Reggie. So we go through only a few drills, and Coach Talbert lets us leave practice before long. The newspaper has a big front-page headline about the death of Reggie and his two brothers, Vaughn, sixteen, and Niarchos, eleven. Over the next few days, Shaw High School seems quiet and sedate. The electricity that usually fills the courtyard during lunch break is missing. The two older Brooks boys were students at Shaw and each was extremely popular. Most of the talk, however, is about Niarchos. People want to know how the father could shoot his youngest son. Maybe Reggie and Vaughn fought him to take up for their mother, people would say. But what could that little eleven-year-old boy have done to that man?

The only credible information anyone really has is in the two newspapers, the morning *Plain Dealer* and the afternoon *Press*. News accounts say that Reginald Brooks Sr. was despondent because his wife planned to divorce him and because he was unemployed. The assistant county coroner is quoted as saying two of the boys were shot from within a few inches and a third boy was slain with a bullet fired from just a few inches farther. School attendance is sparse the day of the funeral, as hundreds of students attend the services at the House of Wills Funeral Home near the projects where Calvin used to live. I decide not to go to the funeral. I don't think I'd be able to handle it, even if I didn't know the victims that well.

The death helps me to begin putting my life in perspective. I start to think about how Reggie would never be able to go to college, get married and have children, or have that National Football League career for which we all thought he was destined. He wouldn't be able to play pick-up basketball or attend concerts. He wouldn't be able to sit back on lazy days and just while away time, like I so often do.

I am thinking that perhaps God is sending a message to me and all my other friends who are not doing much with our lives.

⬛

By the summer of 1982, Natalie and I have pooled our resources and bought an eight-year-old Matador. It is red, with white stripes and a mix-matched yellow hood. After the crash of my Chevy, we need some wheels and this is all we can afford. She and I, both about to enter our senior year, are making business decisions together like a married couple. We buy lunch together every day and now have a car together.

One day that summer, I am driving the Matador through the parking lot on the corner of Brightwood Avenue. Rip Rob is sitting on a railing on the corner and is trying to get my attention. It is dark, hot, and muggy, a typical Cleveland night that time of year.

Hey, Bray! Rip Rob shouts. My music is on but not blaring.

I point the car in his direction and head over. He meets me when I get out.

You seen Bill?

Rip Rob has something else on his mind, something more than just trying to figure out where my Uncle Bill had gone.

Wanna git a wine? he asks.

I'm broke, I tell him.

Rob is jet black, resembling more a Jamaican than a black American. He has a slim runner's body. He is no more than 135 pounds, about five-foot-nine. On a summer night like this, he always wears his shirt unbuttoned, showing off bony chest. He has a short Afro and burning red eyes and a pencil-thin mustache.

I only got about a buck fitty, he says.

We need two mo dollars, I say. A fifth of Wild Irish Rose costs $3.50. We need a fifth because the way the two of us drink, a pint wouldn't bust a grape.

Shit, I know where all the money is, Rob says, smiling. I done hit it once and we can hit it again.

What's up, player, what you talkin' about? I ask.

Church's. We can hit 'em up.

I listen as Rob spells out his plan. I am seventeen. He is about twenty-four. I am waiting for school to start later that year, ready to begin twelfth grade. Rob is a high-school dropout who has already done several prison stints. He lives every day as if it is his last. He is a thief, a robber, a dope fiend, a wino, not trustworthy, and, at the same time, a friend of mine. Actually, he is my Uncle Bill's close friend. But I like hanging out with older guys and have been tailing Bill, Rob, and several other older guys around since I was thirteen. That's the age they started letting me drink wine with them and hanging out over on the strip on Superior Avenue.

We can snatch some dough out of the cash register, Rob says. Just go through the drive-thru, order some food, and when the girls go to git it, just reach your hand in there and take the money.

Both Rob and I have had a few drinks already and are feeling a bit tipsy, but not enough to just call it a night and go home, wherever he calls home these days. Normally, I would have dismissed such a suggestion, but now I am intrigued. I'm not trying to build a name for myself as someone who can pull off a robbery. Just the opposite.

You down? Rob asks.

So you want me to go through the drive-thru, make an order, and when she go to git it, snatch the money?

It's a sure thing, he says confidently.

Man, I heard the police is watchin' that place.

It's Sunday night, Bray. Ain't no damn cops around there.

Let's roll, I say, agreeing to the heist.

We hop into the Matador and within minutes I am talking into the speaker in the drive-thru at Church's. The lights around the restaurant are white-hot bright.

Welcome to Church's. May I take your order? says the voice from the box.

Yeah, you can, I say. Give me, um, give me, um, um. A two-piece, white meat. Some fries and some okra.

Of course, I don't have the money. The voice in the box, a young lady in her late teens, has a latch on the window to prevent robberies. She must think I have a trusting face because she does not lock the window when she goes for my food. The cash drawer is there for me to get to it. I still need to open my door, stick my hand through the window, and try to open the register quickly. I'm not sure I can reach the register but Rob is egging me on.

Gone ahead, make yo move. Now!

I open the door, ease out of the car ever so slightly so that the girl and the other workers inside won't notice my movements. I place my left hand on the silver counter and inch toward the window.

Hurry up, Rob says, a smile crossing his face.

I am now fully out of the car. The door is open even wider. The girl is stuffing chicken and okra into the little white snack box. Rob is egging me on. My heart is pounding fast. I am perspiring but still moving in the right direction.

Suddenly, I jumped back into the car without reaching my hand into the register. Fuck this. I ain't no stick-up man, I say.

I slam the door and speed off, never looking back at the girl who is at the window with my chicken.

Rob is flipping out. What the fuck, Bray? You had it. You had it.

I ain't had nothin', man, making a right out of the restaurant lot and speeding down Superior. We need two fucking dollars, and we are going to rob a place for it. Rob, I say, that ain't for me, man. I ain't no stick-up man.

You ain't got to be. The shit is all set up for yo ass. All you had to do is stick your hand in the window and the dough is there.

Hey, I'll call Natalie's mother. She'll loan my ass five dollars.

Which she did. We somehow manage to get a fifth of Wild Irish Rose and a six-pack of Mickey's Big Mouth malt liquor.

We pull back on Brightwood. I back the Matador into our driveway, with the front end sticking out on the sidewalk. I turn on the Quiet Storm radio program, and Rob and I listen to classic hits and drink our alcohol. He seems to have already forgotten our brief fling with crime, but I am still shaking.

East Cleveland, by any gauge, is a full-fledged ghetto by 1982, the second year into Judge Mosely's six-year term. The once middle-class suburb now has the second highest concentration of black residents in the country behind East St. Louis, Illinois. Murders, rapes, and felonious assaults are up, as well as robberies and house break-ins. Senior citizens are installing thick steel bars over their doors and windows to keep out the hooligans. Empty wine, liquor, and beer bottles are strewn across busy streets, and cars nearly crash into one another trying to prevent their next flat tire. Homes are being abandoned, and no one is enforcing housing-code violations.

As acting judge for four years before his election, Mosely has the petty criminals and neglectful homeowners on the run. With Mosely in town, everyone knows that now offenses such as disturbing the peace with loud music or shooting dice or failing keep up property will surely result in thirty days behind bars and at least a five-hundred-dollar fine. East Cleveland had spun out of control on the watch of the previous judge, who was known for passing out lenient sentences such as Bible reading and essay writing. Not the bespectacled Fred Mosely, who has a round face and wears a 1970s-styled Afro in the era of the Gheri Curl.

Mosely knows East Cleveland well. He moved to the city in the mid-1960s and had been a community activist before becoming an elected official. He has always thought some people bought houses in East Cleveland even though they didn't have the money or the inclination to keep them up. Considering many of East Cleveland's homes were built at the turn of the century, many were in need of major repairs by the time

Mosely took office, if not before. Mosely has put the fear of God even into Grandma.

I betta start fixing up my house before that ol' inspector comes around here again. You know Judge Mosely just trying to get our money, she says.

Mosely has an even bigger effect on some of the city's young criminals who hang out on Brightwood. Most of the young car thieves, stick-up men, and dope dealers don't like talking much about the police or other government officials. They believe if you talk about the cops, the cops come around. On several occasions when I would mention the police, I would be immediately scolded.

Everyone, even my friends who are criminals, talks about Judge Mosely and his style. They contend he is handing out high fines so he can pocket the money. I don't know what to think. I am afraid of the East Cleveland jail and don't want to ever end up in it.

Mosely doesn't like my Uncle Bill very much, either. Bill can't seem to stay out of trouble, and Mosely keeps him locked up for long stretches. Even Bill now tells me he longs for the old days of the former judge, who was more prone to give lectures than tough sentences.

The people who think Fred Mosely, the law-and-order judge, is too good to be true turn out to be right. Three years into his term, Mosely, along with several other city officials, is indicted on a half dozen felony counts of taking kickbacks.

I begin following every detail of the case in the *Cleveland Plain Dealer*. I am fascinated by the work of reporter George Jordan, who digs into the allegations and the reactions by people in East Cleveland. His work seems fun, challenging. I can't believe the level of detail in his stories and how Jordan is able to sum up everything so the average person can understand it.

For the first time I know that I want to go to college and become a newspaper reporter. As for Judge Mosely, he would end up receiving a twelve-year prison sentence.

◩

Grandma and Leroy have taken a trip to Mississippi to visit Leroy's sister. Leroy had left the cotton fields of Mississippi when he was a teen for the freedom of the North. Leroy hates Mississippi and vows never to move back South, even though Grandma talks about returning home to her native Alabama some day.

Boy, it took me too long to git from down there, Bray, Leroy tells me whenever I encourage him and Grandma to leave Cleveland for the slower pace of the South.

Why would I go back? he asks.

Those white folks down there treated me b-a-a-a-d, boy, he says, drawing out the word bad as if he were purging demons by emphasizing it so thoroughly. I work those fields all day long, Bray. Pay me nuthin'. Wouldn't even let me go to school, Bray. Treat me like dirt, boy. I ain't never, ever goin' back down there, you hear me. Other than fo a vacation. You can tell yo grandma to forgit it. Hear me, boy! Tell her to forgit it!

He laughs knowingly, mostly to amuse himself, I suppose.

I come up here. Got me a job at the cah place, cleaning out cahs. Got me a cah, a place to stay, some clothes, good food. Why would I wanna go back, Bray?

He laughs once more.

He goes back and visits, however. And on occasions like this, when Leroy and Grandma are in the South, their home on Brightwood is transformed into a neighborhood hang out. A place to drink beer and use the telephone and

THE GIFT

watch television and play loud music and cards.

That's why Rico is sitting on the porch, busting the cap off a Mickey's Big Mouth. He raises the green, twelve-ounce bottle to his mouth, and the malt liquor flows down his throat. Where the wine? Tom asks.

Dead soldier, Rico says, wiping beer from his chin.

Rico killed it, I say, handing Tom a Big Mouth.

That yo cousin, Bray, Rico says. A shiny blue Oldsmobile, with one-inch white walls, pulls to the curb across the street. Out gets a large and bearded man fashionably dressed in designer shorts and a series of gold chains around his neck.

Whaddup, Jerome? I ask.

Hey, Dwayne, Jerome, my mother's first cousin, says.

Goddam, Jerome says, looking at Rico. You betta git you some new teeth. (I can feel the pain that is about to erupt in my side from the laughter.) Look at them motherfuckers, Jerome says. That ain't plaque is it?

You a funny sonofabitch, I say.

I ain't funny, Dwayne, he says. If I am so damn funny I wouldn't be working for the white man.

Jerome *is* funny. He is born with the gift to make people laugh, and whenever he shows up everybody knows it's time to laugh. But you have to be careful because, like Rico, you never know if Jerome is going to shine the spotlight on you.

Uncle Son walks out on the porch in his boxer shorts, with the fly open. Unc takes his right hand, lifts his boxers in the back and scratches. His fingernails, long as always, make a harsh scratching sound against his leg. They leave long white scratch marks.

Jerome, Unc says, let me git two dollars.

God, Unc, ain't they still paying you black ass up at the car wash? Jerome asks.

Yeah, Unc says. But I don't get paid till Tuesday.

Here you go Unc, Rico says. He pulls out two wrinkled dollars. Unc retreats into the house to get his pants, shirt, and shoes.

Jerome goes into the house to use the phone. Antmo's girlfriend Denise is inside pleading with Andre, Dorothy's son, to take a bath. Andre is resisting, saying he's not ready to bathe. He is six years old and already doing what he wants, already street-hardened.

I ain't taking no bath right now, he insists. Leave me alone.

But Denise is in charge of him tonight.

Rico and Tom have gone into the house. We're about to watch a preseason football game. We sit in the living room and turn on the television.

Denise is still having trouble with Andre.

What's the problem? I ask, knowing full well what it is.

I tell Andre to get in the tub, and he tells me I ain't taking no bath right now.

I lift him up from around the midsection, drape him over my shoulders, and sit him down in the pink chair next to the tub.

Now, you're taking a bath, you hear me?

Jerome the Jokester witnesses this scene. He is not joking now. He starts yelling at me.

You wanna make someone take a bath, you get your own kids, Dwayne.

Hey, Jerome, I made him take a bath, that's all.

He ain't yo kid, Dwayne. You ain't got no business putting yo hands on him at all. Not picking him up or nothing like that.

Look, Romey, I say. I'm here with him every day. I keep him whenever his mother wants to go out. I take him to the store. I spend time with him. You don't come over here once or twice a month and tell me what to do with him.

Like I say, Jerome snaps, keep yo hands off him.

Like I say, Romey, you keep out of it.

He walks over to me, all 250 or so pounds of him. I stand up, and we face off. His gut against my chest. He puts his finger in my face. I hold my head back, away from his pointing finger. All of a sudden I knock his finger out of my face. He pushes me down, back in the chair from which I had risen. He then grabs me by my shirt, tearing it. He has a hold of me, and he is too strong for me to break loose.

I punch him in the face, once, twice, three times.

I know I'm about to get clocked. He tries to lift me off the ground but I resist, so he just throws me down. My cousin has me in a headlock on the floor of Grandma's living room and we are wrestling but he's mostly on top. I manage to get in another punch and by then he's had it. He swings on me and hits me a couple times.

Rico and Tom—my homies, my road dogs who will stick with me through thick and thin—leave. They get up and leave me with this big bear on top of me.

The altercation lasts a couple more minutes. I'm in tears.

He gets up. His fine clothes are now disheveled and torn. He is breathing heavily, which, to me, is a mild victory of sorts. We holler at each other. He picks up his keys, goes out the front door. I hear him pull off.

I'm still sobbing. This is the first time I can remember actually crying in years.

I pick up the phone. Where's my numbers? I say. Denise is trying to stay clear of me.

She finds my phone book. Here, Dwayne.

We have a rotary phone. Big Calvin moved his family

back to Cleveland a few months earlier. I slowly dial seven numbers.

Calvin, I say to Little Calvin, where's your daddy?

Big Cal picks up the phone.

Big Cal, I say, still bawling, barely able to get the words out. That motherfucker Jerome, our cousin, jumped me, man. You got some heat?

◪

I'm sitting on the porch on Brightwood, my sobs down to just a sniffle. Up in the driveway pulls Big Cal. He's driving the five-year-old Mercedes he bought Little Calvin. Little Calvin is in the passenger seat. They both get out of the car slowly, as cool as they want to be. Big Calvin comes over and gives me a big hug. Little Calvin hugs me. I tell them what happens and Big Calvin seems to be getting mad.

No motherfucker puts their hands on you, cousin or no cousin, he says. Get in, he says to me. Calvin, you get in the back, and Dwayne, you up front.

We obey.

Big Calvin goes to the trunk, grabs a bag, and gets in the driver's seat. He pulls out a silver .38. Let's find his ass, Big Calvin says.

I'm taking care of business, I say, meaning I want to shoot Jerome.

Don't worry about that, Big Calvin says. Where he hang out at?

At the Meeting Place over on Hayden, I say. Big Calvin points the Mercedes in that direction and heads forward.

The Meeting Place is a bar in a seedy district on the north side of East Cleveland. The sign says men have to be thirty and older to enter and women at least twenty-five and older. Most of the patrons are working class, like Jerome, a foreman at a Cleveland steel plant. They come home at 5 or 6 P.M., bathe or shower, and slip into their finest threads. They dab on cologne, sprinkle on fragrance, and go out to get the feeling of importance that has eluded them during the workday. It is a dark place, with a long ornamental bar that stretches from one end of the room to the other. You either sit at the bar, as I often had alongside Jerome, or you sat at one of the dozen tables or so in the back of it.

Big Calvin slips the pistol into his waist, tells his son to stay in the car, and orders me into the bar. Find Jerome, he says, and let me know when you see him. I am sure Jerome has gone to the Meeting Place for a drink after our altercation. I go inside and sidle up to the bar. My eyes are red from crying but I am composed. Teddy, Jerome's brother and perhaps my favorite older male cousin in the world, is at the bar.

Hey, Ted, I say.

He is three sheets to the wind. What's up? he says.

You seen Jerome? I say.

Earlier, he says.

Calvin and I hit a couple more bars on the far East Side of East Cleveland. Jerome is nowhere to be found. But Calvin keeps driving. I don't realize that, by now, he's only driving to calm me down.

He goes up Forest Hills Boulevard and heads over to Coventry Street. We go into a Thai food restaurant. In no time, I'm eating and smiling and laughing. I'm with Big

Calvin and Little Calvin and have stopped thinking about my fight with Jerome.

But I haven't stopped thinking about Rico and Tom. They were supposed to have had my back.

PART

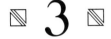 3

Most of the guys I hang around with are high-school dropouts. They are loyal to our turf, but they steal cars, sell dope, and spend most days whiling away their lives in what seems to the larger world to be useless pursuits. To them and to me, this is the best they can do, given the inferior education we all received in East Cleveland public schools, where the teachers oftentimes were more interested in keeping the peace than feeding the mind. I've managed to procure a diploma, with the help of my girlfriend, Natalie, and a few special teachers who were determined not to let the streets devour me. But the fact is, I am barely a high-school grad, graduating with a low C average.

Even with such poor grades, Cleveland State is bound to accept me as a student because it is a publicly funded state university charged with educating anyone who has earned a diploma from an accredited Ohio school system.

One day, my close friend Don says, That's pretty good, you finishing school. You hang around the streets like these other motherfuckas and you don't see any of them graduating. But you did. That's something to be proud of.

Graduating felt good. It was an achievement. The odds, given my self-selected peer group, were heavily against me. But while I now know that I will get a fresh start on my GPA in college, I am more proud that Don notices my work and effort, and that he acknowledges my accomplishment. Most of my friends pooh-pooh academics. Going to school is a sign of weakness to them, not something to wear around one's neck like a badge of honor.

I never doubted finishing high school. My mother, despite her drug addiction, is smart and relatively well read. So why shouldn't the same be true of me?

◨

Grandma still gets a welfare check to take care of me. It's called AFDC, for Aid to Families with Dependent Children. I'm eighteen, finished high school, and unemployed. It's the summer of 1983, and I will be attending Cleveland State University in the fall. For some reason, probably because I have my eyes set on moving out of the house and somehow getting my own apartment, I decide Grandma should no longer draw welfare for me. So shortly before school is set to begin, I catch the bus downtown to the Department of Human Resources to get the check switched over to my own name. Grandma doesn't know what I'm up to.

I am familiar with the welfare office. I've come here many times with both my mother and Grandma. It is still located at 220 St. Clair Avenue, the same place it was when I was born, and Grandma had to come argue with the caseworker for increased benefits in order to keep me. It is a busy place with people lined up at different windows, people sitting in waiting rooms reading the paper and smoking cigarettes. People, mothers mostly, trying to control unruly kids. These women wait up to two and three hours just to talk to someone about their benefits. It's tough to keep a kid still for that long.

I take a seat next to a heavyset lady with kids ranging from a few months old to about six or seven. These children are crawling under chairs, sliding on the tile floor, fighting with one another. She tries her best to calm them down, but she and the rest of us realize how futile this is.

I am ashamed of being here. I look around and feel sorry for some of these people. Many look ragged and are chain-smoking. Some don't even have front teeth. Most of them talk without using proper English. I feel guilty because I am thinking they belong here and I don't. They are here because they are irresponsible. These women have had babies out of wedlock. These men have dropped out of school and abused drugs and alcohol and women. I have not really done any of that. I am a high school graduate who is about to start college. I have not fathered any illegitimate children. I want to work, but the only job available is my seasonal peanut-selling gig. I am here because my mother is a junkie, not because I belong here. I try to distinguish myself by reading the business section of the newspaper. I look at the stock tables, even though I have no idea what I'm reading. I want people to believe I'm smart.

Finally, after a wait of about an hour, my name is called. I am told that before I can sign up for General Relief, which is the benefit program for able-bodied males, I must first have Grandma's AFDC check cut off. I think, She's going to kill me for cutting off her benefits.

But I am grown, and she should not be getting benefits for me any longer. So I head to the third floor, wait another couple of hours, and terminate Grandma's

AFDC. Then it's off to another floor, where I finally get to the General Relief line. I am still embarrassed for being here and eager to tell the caseworker that, indeed, I am a high school graduate and I am enrolled at Cleveland State in hopes of earning a degree and becoming a journalist. I am one client who really wants to get off welfare.

The caseworker just nods and tells me that I will receive a check for $108 a month, which is the same amount Grandma receives for my care. The only difference is the check will now come to me, not her. Grandma also gets more than $100 a month in food stamps and, to my total shock, the caseworker says that the state of Ohio will no longer provide me with food stamps.

What? Why? I need those stamps to eat, I explain.

It's because you're enrolled in college, Mr. Bray, she says.

But you don't understand—I have to eat.

Get your grandmother to feed you, she suggests.

But my grandmother uses those food stamps to feed me, I tell her.

Well, you should have kept your benefits in her name, the woman says derisively. She is telling me that I would have been better off keeping the benefits in Grandma's name, even though I'm now grown and am under obligation to report this fact.

I ask the woman, If I go down to Cleveland State, drop out, and just hang around my old neighborhood all day without working, you mean to tell me that *then* you will give me food stamps?

That's the system, Mr. Bray, the woman says. You see, Mr. Bray, a lot of college students from well-off families try to use the system to get food stamps just to party with. To stop that abuse, the state decided to cut all college students off food stamps. You're just a victim of that. Sorry.

I leave thinking how upset Grandma is going to be when she discovers what I have done. But I know that Grandma can never stay mad at me for long. She has strong spiritual faith and, like Job, is as patient as they come. And she really wants to be patient with me. Grandma interfered in my Uncle Bill's life in the late '70s, after he got out of the army and wanted to be a police-man. She convinced him that line of work was dangerous and, after briefly taking up mechanical drafting, he set-tled into a life of crime. Grandma wrongly blamed herself for Bill's predicament, and she vowed never again to interfere with her kids' or grandkids' decisions.

I am right. Grandma isn't happy with me when I inform her that I have managed to get our food stamps cut off. I tell her it doesn't matter much anyway, that as soon as school starts in the fall, I plan to find a job. She gets over her anger with me and begins to focus on a system that denies food stamps to an unemployed young man just because he is enrolled in college trying to get an education to pull himself up by his bootstraps.

I spend every day in the summer of 1983 stuck in the same routine, and it all starts with Uncle Son around eight in the morning. Unc has credit with Nip, the owner of the corner store. Every morning at 8 A.M. when Nip's opens, Unc is their first customer. He adds to his tab a pack of Pall Malls, a twelve-pack of Olde English 800 malt liquor, and a fifth of Wild Irish Rose. Unc is like Mama, his sister: free-hearted. He believes in sharing. When he returns from the store, he lights up a cigarette and comes to the room where Antmo and I are sleeping.

Y'all boys better come on before I drink all this stuff up, he says.

Antmo always jumps up, throws on his clothes and goes downstairs where the spirits are. He reaches into the brown paper sack, pulls out a tall-boy can of malt liquor and takes a long drink. Usually I follow the same routine. We either sit at the kitchen table or out on the front porch in three chairs lined together. We talk and wave at the people passing, some going to work, others heading to the store to buy something to drink themselves.

Unc is walking up the street fast today. It is 8:15 in the morning, and he has his daily allowance of a twelve-pack of malt liquor, a fifth of wine, and a pack of cigarettes. Antmo and I are sitting on the porch, waiting to grab a beer and start off our day. I am wearing only a pair of white cutoffs. No shirt, no shoes, no socks.

Damn, Unc, I say before he reaches our driveway. You forgot the paper.

Sho did, he says.

In addition to beer and wine, I have gotten used to starting off my day by reading the morning newspaper. Unc apologizes, takes a seat, and pulls out a six-pack of the tall boys of Olde English.

Here, Bray, he says, handing me one of the cold brown cans. Antmo reaches over and tears a can apart from the plastic holder. We sit and drink and talk about things that aren't really important. Unc scoots his chair back and forth for no reason and then busts out in a loud, spontaneous laugh.

Cocksucker, motherfucker, kiss my black ass! he hollers. Laura B., Laura B., Laura B., he says, calling out the name of my dead aunt Laura.

Antmo and I are used to his outbursts, and we just

keep drinking. Then Unc makes a staccato sound. *Tack, tack, tack, tack, tack, tack.* He keeps repeating the same sound.

Finally, Antmo has had enough. He walks over to him and puts a hand on his shoulder. Cut that shit out, Mo says to our uncle.

Unc has a cigarette in his hand and he just looks down at it with a steely gaze, taking his right thumb and rubbing directly over the fire at the cigarette's tip. He is ignoring Antmo who is still standing above him with a hand on his shoulder.

I am watching my two uncles, one crazy, the other trying to calm him down. I turn around toward the street at the sound of my name. It is Pokey. He is headed to the store, for what I don't know.

Hey, Poke, I call out. Can you pick me up a newspaper?

I get up to get him some change to buy the paper, but he waves me off and says he'll pay for it. Everyone in the neighborhood knows I like to sit on the front porch and read the paper. I sit there and wait for Pokey to return. Unc is calm now, asking me about Cleveland State—if I'm scared of the courses, do I think I can handle the work. We drink and talk about higher education, something none of us has ever experienced. Before long, Pokey is back with the newspaper. I unfold it and plastered across the front page is this headline: Man Found Dead at Cleveland State.

The story says that a black man was found dead in a bathroom at the university.

I look over to Unc, point to the story, and say, Hell yeah, I'm scared to go to Cleveland State.

By the time I arrive on campus at Cleveland State, Frank Spisak, the murderer, has been arrested and charged with killing three people, including two blacks. A white supremacist and neo-Nazi, he is later convicted and sentenced to die. With Spisak behind bars, I plan on concentrating on my studies. I am placed in special studies, a program for academically weak students that is designed to help prepare me for entrance into the College of Arts & Sciences, where I can major in communication and pursue a career as a newspaper reporter.

It doesn't take me long to realize that most of my special studies classmates are black. Most of us come from the innercity school systems of Cleveland and East Cleveland and are so far behind that we need classes like basic math, basic reading, and basic English.

During my second quarter in the winter of 1984, I receive unsatisfactory grades in Eng 098, the lowest-level English class offered at Cleveland State, and in Math 100, a class so low that even when you pass it you don't receive credit for the work. I am seriously considering whether I should even be in college and come close to just dropping out.

But by now, I have joined the *Vindicator*, the twice-monthly black student newspaper. I enjoy writing sports articles for the paper, but know that my grades are so poor I should be concentrating full-time on my studies. Instead, I continue spending most of my days reading the *Cleveland Plain Dealer* and working on my own stories—things I enjoy and am good at. I go to class but basically don't pay much attention to the instructors. I want to learn, I want to do well, but my study habits are so poor that I can't overcome my own inadequacies.

My classes are on Tuesdays and Thursdays. I spend the other five days of the week hanging around Brightwood with Unc and Antmo and Pokey and my other friends. We drink beer, shoot dice, play cards, and just have ourselves a merry old time. When school time comes, I get up and go, like I always have, but I am of course not prepared.

☒

I know I need to take classes in the summer of 1984. I have just finished my first full year at Cleveland State and my grade-point average is 2.18. The unsatisfactory grades I received in special studies don't count against my average and in six other classes I receive five Cs and one B. Those grades come not because I studied but because I was smart enough to pass them without studying. The grades also show me that if I study and quit hanging out with high-school dropouts all the time, I probably could do better for myself.

One day that summer, I am hanging out with Poochie, a third cousin. We are at the Taylor apartments at the corner of Taylor and Terrace. I should be at home studying, but we are cruising East Cleveland. Poochie is having a problem with his live-in girlfriend. I pull up in the parking lot of their apartment building, and Poochie gets out of the car and goes inside.

I am sitting in my latest car, a Dodge Duster, all painted gold, when I hear some arguing. I get out of the car to see what it is, and see Poochie in the corridor standing face to face with two men. One of the men pushes my cousin, and he goes flying into a wall. I dash over, screaming that Poochie is my cousin and that these men will have to take on the two of us.

I go directly for the man who has pushed Poochie. He takes a wild swing at me in this cramped apartment hallway. I dodge the punch and throw one of my own. I connect, and the man, in his late twenties, goes flying against the wall. We face off but no more punches are thrown.

I don't wanna fight you, man, he says.

Poochie's girlfriend is in the doorway looking out. These men are with her, maybe her relatives.

Poochie and I walk out of the building, never turning our backs on the men.

N

I have had enough. My grades stink, I am hanging out with high-school dropouts who can't keep a job, and now I am getting into street fights more frequently.

Natalie and I have been arguing. She knows my life isn't going right and so do I, but I'm in denial about almost everything. I won't admit the crowd I'm hanging around with is bad news. I won't admit that one of these days, one of the men in the hallways or on the street corners with whom I scuffle is going to pull out a gun and blow my brains away. My grandmother repeats this all the time: Dwayne, stay out of trouble. Go to school, boy, and get yoself an education. Okay?

Gradually, some of that begins to soak in. And I have a solution.

N

It is late April 1984, and Natalie and I are talking. We are sitting on her mother's sofa.

Look, I say. I know I can do better, but we have to work together.

She has heard it all before, and I think she is tiring of my old sorry line.

Let's get married, I say.

She looks at me and can't believe I'm serious. She's mad at me anyway about something or other I've done.

She doesn't believe me or she's too angry with me to respond. She waits and waits, and I beg and beg.

Finally, she says yes.

You have to tell my father, she says.

We are sitting on Natalie's couch and her father, Nat, is standing before us. He has a big green apple in one hand and a pocketknife in the other. He is peeling the apple, and I tell him I have something to say.

Go on, he orders me.

Uh, Mr. Williams, I say. Uh, we are getting married.

Mr. Williams just continues to carve up that apple. He stands above us, knife in hand. He doesn't say anything, he doesn't even look at me. He is focused on that apple and then finally he says, Oh yeah?

Uh, yeah, I say.

I think he likes me, but he also knows I grew up on Brightwood and that I have a wild side.

He asks us how we arrived at this decision and what our plans are. He wants to know when we plan on doing this. We tell him October.

Dwayne, he says, looking at me with the knife in his hand, whatever you do, don't hit my daughter.

I don't look at him. I look at his knife.

I won't, I say.

◣

October 6, 1984, comes fast. Natalie and I have saved our money and get all we can from her father and Grandma for our wedding. My big worry is whether my mother is going to make it up from Houston. She said she would. The last time I talked with her, she was out of prison and said she was doing well, relatively speaking.

But she doesn't make it and she doesn't call, either. She's back in jail, stealing to support her drug habit. She misses my wedding, just like she missed my high-school graduation.

On our wedding day, Burning Bush Church is well decorated. I am standing in front of the crowded church with Don, the guy whom I hang out with the most in the hood and who is my best man. Antmo and Calvin and Bobby are in the wedding party, but not my mother's older brother, Bill. He, too, is in prison. Natalie has picked my Aunt Dorothy and two friends, Rita and Stacey, to be in the wedding. The wedding goes off without a hitch and, afterward, the wedding party rides around Cleveland drinking champagne in a rented limousine before the reception.

We go over to Brightwood and over to Woodlawn, a couple streets away. The wedding party poses for pictures at a big lake behind Severance Hall. The reception is in the party room of a somewhat seedy downtown motel, but that's all we can afford. With the party in full bloom, bride and groom leave. We have a room awaiting us in the honeymoon suite of the Sheraton Hotel in downtown Cleveland. A bottle of champagne awaits us. Natalie doesn't drink, so I pour her some pop and myself some champagne. We open our gifts, including several hundred dollars in cash. We can't afford a real, out-of-the-country honeymoon, but we vow that one day we will be successful and go on the trip of our lives.

◪

Married life doesn't turn me into a scholar, not right away at least. During the academic quarter before the wedding, with all the planning and all the nervousness, my grade point average dips to 1.88. Getting married only puts more stress on my time. I now need to work, and I get a job as a cashier at McDonald's. I help open up the downtown store, work until noon, and then go to class.

For a while after becoming a husband, I quit hanging out so much and partying with my childhood friends and my relatives. But that doesn't last long. At school, I apply for a job that will give me actual work experience. I tell the counselor I want to work at the *Plain Dealer*, Cleveland's daily newspaper, the same paper I have read religiously for years. I am thinking I will get a position in the newsroom as a clerk, helping the reporters and editors. After all, I am now sports editor of the *Vindicator,* and the newsroom training at the *Plain Dealer* would do more to help my future career in journalism than anything else.

The good news is that I land a position at the *Plain Dealer.* The bad news is that it isn't in the newsroom. Instead, I am hired at Cleveland's daily newspaper as a customer-service representative. I have no contact with reporters and editors. I get in early in the morning and take complaints and other requests from customers. The job pays more than seven dollars an hour, but it is only for six months.

A week after I begin work, one of the supervisors walks by my desk and hands me a gray envelope. It is my paycheck. I open it, and it's for more than two hundred dollars. I am pleased that Uncle Sam didn't hit me up for too much in taxes.

At lunch break, I dash out of the building and catch a twenty-five-cent loop bus that takes me to the Ameritrust Bank on the corner of Euclid and Ninth streets. I stand in line waiting to cash my first paycheck. The bank is huge and there are maybe a dozen teller windows operating. I plan to get my money and head over to my favorite deli for a thick corned-beef sandwich before my break is up.

All the teller windows are moving fast except the one I'm at. I've been at the window for five minutes or longer and the teller keeps stalling. What's wrong? I ask. We just have to verify the check, she says.

Verify? I shoot back. It's the *Plain Dealer*. You know, that newspaper that's been around for a hundred years. They're not going bankrupt.

Suddenly, I am surrounded by a half dozen armed guards.

Mr. Bray, my name is Parkowski, and I'm in charge of bank security. Can you follow me?

Parkowski is a no-nonsense cop. He has a battery of bouncer-type guards with him, so I follow.

What's the problem? I ask innocently.

Just follow, Parkowski says.

They take me to a corner of the bank. Parkowski is carrying my check. I am seated in a chair, and the armed guards hover over me.

Sir, you have been identified as someone who possibly robbed this bank once before, Parkowski said.

That's crazy! I exclaim. I'm a college student, and I work in the circulation department over at the *Plain Dealer*. That's my check in your hand.

Parkowski says this is a serious matter and that he's doing some checking.

I beg them to let me call my job, if for nothing else to let them know I will be late getting back from lunch, if I ever get back. They deny my requests. I watch the clock and as it inches toward 1 P.M., the time I am due back to work, I get louder. They agree that I can call.

I tell my supervisor what's going on. Parkowski gets on the phone and informs her that I am a bank-robbery suspect and I am in federal custody. He hangs up.

The checking goes on for another forty-five minutes, and I just sit there under armed guard. Parkowski has been on the phone nonstop and suddenly he hangs up and comes over to me.

You can go now, he says.

What do you mean? I say. What do you mean I can go now? You and Ameritrust have just blown my lunch, held me under arrest, and now that's all you have to say?

One of the bulky guards advises me that I should just leave.

I do so, but not before demanding a business card from Parkowski. He gives me one and doesn't seem very bothered at all about harassing me. His expressions says, No big deal, I'm just doing my job, and if that means inconveniencing one of Ameritrust's customers, who cares, as long as the customer is a young black male and not a middle-aged white male who could take action against my ass.

I am furious. My grandmother suggests I call Mr. Steinberg, her lawyer. But I want Stanley Tolliver, the important black lawyer I see on television wearing the wide-brimmed hats and taking on all the civil-rights cases.

I arrange an appointment with Stanley Tolliver. He hears me out and says, I'm gonna git you some money, young man. They can't do this to you.

Months go by and I never hear from Tolliver. Once, I get him on the phone and he says something about handing the case off to his assistant and the assistant is out of town and he'll check on it when the assistant gets back.

Tolliver never does call back and I let the matter die.

◩

In six months, my stay at the *Plain Dealer* is over. I am hoping they will hire me permanently, like they have some other co-op students. I work hard and show up on time. I'm congenial with the bosses and my coworkers. I am very productive, taking a high rate of customer calls, and get an excellent evaluation. But they let me go, and in the back of my mind, I wonder if the bank incident has anything to do with my not being asked to stay on.

I am now an unemployed student again, which is horrible news because Natalie is pregnant. Natalie is working part-time as a secretary with no benefits. She leaves that job when her due date nears.

I go to school and put in job applications every day. Bobby, my uncle and former roommate, and I land jobs at a local company that sorts mail for the post office. We are hired for $4.75 an hour. I spend my days during the summer of 1985 sorting out mail by hand. Every night my arms are sore from all the sorting. I also get an assignment officiating intramural basketball games at Cleveland State, a job I love but it pays only about seventy-five dollars a week. None of this is enough money for a husband and father-to-be.

In the fall of 1985, I get a call from the *Plain Dealer*. I am hired as a permanent part-time customer service rep for $8.25 an hour. I can also purchase health benefits, which is good considering my first child is due in four months.

On January 25, 1986, after eighteen hours of labor, Natalie gives birth to our son, Dwayne Bray Jr. I am in the delivery room at Booth Memorial Hospital on Cleveland's East Side. It is Super Bowl Sunday and the Chicago Bears, behind running back Walter (Sweetness) Payton, are on the TV monitor beating up on the New England Patriots, 46 to 10.

Fatherhood does more to settle me down, for a while at least, than anything else, including marriage. Dwayne Jr. is awesome. He is little and has curly hair. Natalie is afraid of crib death, so he sleeps with us. With Dwayne Jr. in the house, I stop spending so much time after school and after work on Brightwood. Instead, I invite my buddies down to my apartment, under the rationalization that at least I'm at home when I hang out with them, drinking beer, either watching a ball game or on the porch cooking out.

Natalie realizes I am trying hard to be a father, never having known one of my own. She also knows I'm trying to be a good husband and provider and tolerates, for the most part, my urges to hang around with my friends from before our marriage.

I spend most of my time with Don, the best man at our wedding. He is an intelligent guy who, like most of my buddies in East Cleveland, dropped out of high school. His daughter, Sierra, is born shortly after my son. But Don and Sierra's mother, Valerie, split up. So Don is single, and I am married, and that is a bad combination.

When Don and I are not hanging around, I'm usually with Poochie. He learned the printing business when he was in the army and is now a journeyman printer. He likes to drink a lot and misses work often and is frequently fired. But he has a marketable trade, so he usually lands on his feet.

One summer night Poochie and I hit every bar in East Cleveland until they are all closed. We then eat at a late-night Polish Boy restaurant and head to my house at 4 A.M. Natalie refuses to let us in, one of the few times she has shown such defiance.

When I am not hanging out, I am usually at the *Plain Dealer*, stopping and starting vacationers' newspapers or directing the district manager truck drivers to their next drop-off site.

At school, I am still making C grades, which isn't great but moves me closer to graduation. I have also crossed over to write for the *Cauldron*, the main campus newspaper. Leaving the *Vindicator*, which dealt mostly with issues that affected blacks on campus, was a difficult decision. Sometimes I think that in some small way I am blazing a trail for other blacks by crossing over to the *Cauldron*. Maybe that's why I'm confused about the move. I am saying it's okay for blacks to write for a paper that has traditionally had mostly white writers and editors. This doesn't compare to the ground broken by Jackie Robinson, mind you, but in my small world it is as deep as it gets.

To the consternation of some staffers at the *Cauldron*, I am named sports editor over at least one staffer who wanted the position. So life seems to be looking up for me: I am sports editor of Cleveland State's main newspaper; I am a father; I am a husband; I am weaning myself off Brightwood and the mean streets of East Cleveland.

◩

All I'm doing is a favor for Bill, my uncle and my mother's oldest brother. He notices some new summer clothes I'm wearing. When I tell him I got this gear at T. J. Maxx in Wickliffe, a suburb about twenty miles east of our neighborhood, he asks if I could give him a lift out there. That next Saturday, I leave my circulation job at the Plain Dealer around noon and pick Bill up at the house on Brightwood. We drive to T. J. Maxx, where Bill does some shopping, buying some jeans, a belt, some shirts, and other clothing articles. I just browse. The store is big and airy. Most of the other customers are white, except for a black guy who appears to be about my age. We nearly bump into each other, and he apologizes.

No problem, bro, I say.

Bill is ready to leave. His shopping cart is full and we make our way toward the check-out counter. The check-out clerk is also black and she chats with us as she rings up Bill's merchandise. The sun beams brightly through the large pane glass window. I pick up a pair of discounted sunglasses on display at the counter. They are only $1.99.

Blood, I say, calling Bill by his street name. Why don't you buy these for me, and we're even for the ride.

You want me to put those in the bag, the cashier says.

Nah, that sun's bright, I say. I'll just wear 'em.

Bills pays and we head out to my car. We are outside the store on the sidewalk when we are suddenly swarmed by about a half dozen people.

Store security, a man in a *Miami Vice* get-up says. Against the wall!

They are talking to me. I protest.

You stole those glasses, the *Miami Vice* wanna-be says.

No, I didn't, I respond angrily. Bill, show 'em the receipt.

I reach for Bill's bag, but the store cop grabs my hand before I can get the receipt. He pushes me against the pane-glass window and the other detectives close in on me. The other black guy I had bumped into inside the store is also spread eagle against the window.

You two are working together, a woman alleges.

I have never seen this guy in my life before today, I say.

They search the other guy and me. They tell him to leave, that they have nothing on him. They tell me that I have stolen the sunglasses for which we have paid. I'm incredulous. They parade me back in the store and Bill tries to follow.

What y'all doing with him? Bill demands.

We're taking him to the office, the woman replies. And you can't go.

Bill, who is six foot five, about 205 pounds, tries to push his way through. I know what y'all do to young black boys back in those rooms—he ain't going nowhere, Bill says, following us through the store.

All these white customers are looking, as if Bill and I are criminals. I manage to slip Bill my car keys so he can drive home. Bill has a prison record and, even though we are totally innocent, I know that if they find out he is an ex-con, we're in bigger trouble.

Here, take these keys and get out of here, I say.

What about you? he says.

I'll be all right, I tell him as the head security guy continues to push me through the store, past all the stares.

Bill is refusing to leave the store because I have been arrested. One of the security guys gets on the phone and calls Wickliffe police. We have a black male shoplifter in custody and we have an accomplice who is unruly, the

officer tells the Wickliffe dispatcher.
Bill hears the call to the cops and leaves.

�– ◆ –

In no time, I hear sirens. I am in the back of the store, alone with the store security personnel, or loss-prevention officers, as they call themselves. About four cops burst through the back door, one with a dog on a leash.

I'm even more incredulous. All I've done today is get up at 4:30 A.M. to be at work by 5 A.M. Worked my ass off and then gave my uncle a ride to this prejudiced hick town. And what do I get for all that? Arrested, accused, pushed around, and, now I'm about to go to jail, escorted by a fucking police dog.

The security guy tells the police officer that I have stolen a pair of sunglasses. I implore the officer to talk to the black cashier. She knows we bought them, I say.

Mr. Bray, calm down, the officer says.

The cashier is not involved in this, the head security guy says. This is a security matter.

Fuck that, I say. She knows first-hand that we paid for those glasses. Just ask her and clear this matter up.

Mr. Bray, will you calm down? the Wickliffe officer says in a stern manner.

Calm down for what? I demand. I haven't done anything.

The officer, a clean-cut white guy in his mid-twenties, says that he has to take me to jail because the loss-prevention officer wants to file a formal complaint of theft. I am handcuffed, stuffed in the back of the cruiser like cargo, and hauled to the Wickliffe police station. There I am photographed just like the criminals on those television police shows; my mug is taken from the front and then left and right profile shots. My fingers are smudged with black ink and my prints are taken.

I get one phone call.

Natalie, I'm in jail, I say.

What?!

Now I'm telling her to calm down. I explain the events and tell her that I have a five-hundred-dollar bond, but that I can be released if she brings fifty dollars to the jail. She hangs up and springs into action.

While I wait on my bail, I am led to a cell. I have always feared being locked up in a jail cell. I do not fear violence from other prisoners; I grew up on Brightwood and learned to defend myself. I am claustrophobic, however, and fear being in tight, cramped quarters.

Wickliffe has two two-man cells. Each one has a double bunk and a sink and toilet. The young officer takes me back to the cells, slips the key in the door of the first one, and opens it. I'm the only prisoner on this Saturday afternoon.

There you go, Mr. Bray, he says. He tells me that if I get my bail I will be released, otherwise I will be in for the entire weekend and will go to court on Monday. I profess my innocence once more and that's when he gets a good look at me.

I've seen your name somewhere, he says. Do you go to Cleveland State?

Yeah, I answer.

I read your articles on the basketball team all the time, he says.

I'm the sports editor of the *Cauldron*, I tell him.

Well, I believe you about those glasses, he says apologetically, but when the store wants to file a complaint, we have to take people to jail. That's how it works out here.

Yeah, I know, I tell him. It's not your fault.

I feel better that he has recognized me. This means he

will treat me well, which he does. He brings me some magazines and tells me to just call out if I need anything else. I don't, because within an hour Natalie has posted my bail and I'm set free. I walk to the car, fresh from the pokey, with my wife and my infant son.

◪

Word spreads quickly around Brightwood that I have been locked up in Wickliffe. Most of the local thugs come to pay me a visit. My brief incarceration becomes a badge of honor.

You don't like that shit, do you schoolboy? Walt Toney says, teasing me. You betta keep yo ass in those books, 'cause they treat you like they wanna in lockup.

Walt should know. Since his teenage years, he has been in and out of corrections institutions of all kinds. But like many other toughs in the neighborhood, Walt wants badly to see someone from here make it out on the strength of their brain. Right now, I'm the favorite and these guys are pulling for me.

◪

There is a saying in our predominantly black community that blacks are good barbers and funeral directors but not good doctors or lawyers. And after my earlier problem with Stanley Tolliver, I am not going to go to a black lawyer to handle my T. J. Maxx case. The man for whom Natalie had worked recommended a lawyer in his building. Bill and I go to see him and he listens to our account of events. The lawyer explains that he will take on the criminal case as a favor to my wife's boss, but he advises me to get a less expensive attorney to handle the civil part of it, if I want to file a lawsuit. In other words, the case isn't big enough for him. There's nothing I can do, so I accept his offer and pay him $475 to get the criminal portion dismissed.

For a civil lawyer, I hire a young Cleveland lawyer who is not long out of law school. He negotiates with T. J. Maxx for nearly eleven months. Eventually, the store agrees to pay me five thousand dollars not to sue. I accept. Natalie and I use our portion of the money to move from East Cleveland to a townhouse in suburban Warrensville Heights. This is a good move because it gets me farther away from some of the negative influences in my life. I am better able to concentrate on work and school during the week, although I can't quite cut the cord—I still spend my weekends hanging out on Brightwood.

My new job as sports editor of the *Cauldron* helps me immeasurably during the 1985-86 school year. All of a sudden, professors who paid no attention to me recognize my name when they call roll at the beginning of each quarter. In one class, a professor calls my name on the first day. I say, Here. He says, Oh, we have a celebrity in our class.

This quarter I am not studying that hard but the professor gives me better grades than I have ever gotten at Cleveland State. I am convinced that as sports editor of the main newspaper, the white newspaper, I am now seen as someone special, someone with leadership qualities.

The flip side is that I think my confidence is shooting up. I am spending less time hanging out in the old neighborhood and more time actually cracking open books to study. The pride of being sports editor of the *Cauldron* is forcing me to work harder in class, not to embarrass the paper and my editor, Nick Kovijanic.

At the *Cauldron*, our big production nights are Sundays and Wednesdays because we publish on Mondays and Thursdays. We all work pretty well together. Nick likes his staff, especially with me editing the sports pages, and a guy from Euclid, Mark Lantz, editing the features pages.

One night, we are all around typesetting copy and laying it out. We are talking about Chicago and I mention something about a trip I once made to Illinois, but I pronounce the word, Ill-e-noise.

It's Ill-i-noi, Nick says.

Well, now I know, I tell him.

That's something you should have known back in elementary school, he says.

For a while, I am seething. His remark is uncalled for, I think. Later, however, on further reflection I realize I am now hanging out with guys who demand excellence, guys who will not allow me to be an underachiever. They are smart and hardworking and headed for bigger and better things in life. And if I'm going to be part of their clique, I need to be smart and hardworking and ambitious as well.

I improve my vocabulary and pronunciation by going to the library and reading *Time* and *Newsweek*. I begin diving into international and national issues of economics and politics and society. I start to broaden my horizons outside the scope of the little ghetto where I grew up. Nick and the others grew up in suburban communities where academics were stressed and the teachers spent time teaching. They had parents who made sure they were in the house at a decent time and that their homework was completed. I had neither that nor the discipline to teach those things to myself. I am just learning the beauty of knowledge.

I also decide to learn more about my own cultural

history. Up to this point, all I really know about blacks is what I've seen on television and in the various communities I've lived, basically East Cleveland and Meridian, Mississippi. Now, however, I take a class in African-American writers with Mwatabu Okantah, an instructor at Cleveland State and director of the African American Cultural Center. We read books by Toni Morrison and Zora Neale Hurston. Most of the students in the class are liberal whites who seem to be mesmerized by Okantah's grasp of his material. With his dreadlocks flowing and dressed in African garb, he is theatrical and very confident. He lectures about the writers, but he also talks about history and how slavery, for instance, affects how blacks live today. One day a white female student starts crying in class and says Okantah seems to be blaming her and her ancestors for all of society's ills. I am captivated by her guilt and the way Okantah refuses to let up on her, even as tears stream down her face. I'm feeling sorry for this girl, not knowing that she is a liberal and apparently is only trying to exorcise some demons. This all seems too much.

Still, I leave some of Okantah's lectures feeling guilty about my lack of knowledge of African-American writers. I feel guilty that I've spent so much time hanging around street corners shooting dice and causing trouble. I feel guilty that everyone back in the old neighborhood thinks I'm so smart, when compared to Okantah or even Nick and Mark, I'm really just a dumb fuck who can't pronounce Illinois and doesn't know his own history. And, of course, with Okantah's lectures spinning through my head, I feel guilty for having abandoned the black student newspaper in favor of a job at the *Cauldron*. What kind of confused black man am I?

For the first time, learning is becoming exciting and

stimulating and, at once, challenging. I am beginning to realize that if I am ever to reach my potential, to master my own cultural history and chosen profession as has Okantah, I will have to devote long hours to studying and conquering the nuances of being a smart person. I have taken baby steps, and they are both painful and pleasurable. It is so delicious soaking up the prose of Maya Angelou, Toni Cade Bambara, Gwendolyn Brooks, Alice Childress, Nikki Giovanni, Carolyn Rodgers, and, of course, Toni Morrison and Alice Walker. I drank up every word of *The Third Life of Grange Copeland* by Walker and Hurston's *Their Eyes Were Watching God*. Maybe the guys on Brightwood with whom I waste so much time know better than I. Maybe they realized that once I truly felt the sensation of learning, I would love it and I would begin to leave them behind. If that's the case, they were right. Maybe they knew my potential long before I did.

◩

In the spring of 1987, I am still 60 hours short of the 192 I need to graduate from Cleveland State. I plan to drop all my outside activities, even my job at the *Cauldron*, to finish school within a year. But somehow, the staff votes unanimously to elect me as the new editor-in-chief of the *Cauldron*, the first black ever to hold the position.

I call my cousin Calvin to tell him of my decision to accept the job, despite the demands it will put on my time. He tells me he's proud of me and that one day it will all pay off and I'm going to be a successful journalist. But Calvin is having some success of his own. And it's in the one area I am most in love with: sports.

Little Calvin is seventeen and lives with his dad, Big Calvin, and his stepmom, Dana, in Cleveland Heights.

When we were kids, only well-off blacks lived in Cleveland Heights but now the city has become more eclectic and 37 percent of its fifty-four thousand residents are black. Because blacks have always striven for achievement in football and basketball—areas where they thought the doors of opportunity were open—the Cleveland Heights teams are the recipients of all this new talent.

Calvin plays football. He is five foot eleven, 185 pounds, and the defensive leader of the Tigers' team. He's seventeen and one of the most popular students at Heights High. He has already taken a recruiting trip to the University of Pitt with some of Cleveland's other top high school recruits, including Desmond Howard, a running back/receiver at St. Joseph's High School and perhaps the top prep football player in Ohio.

Calvin knows that all that could keep him from a big-time college football career, and possibly a shot at playing in the NFL, are academic problems. He is never a great student, but he tells me that he is getting Bs and Cs and is on track to graduate.

I still can't believe he's as good as advertised because no one from our family, except me, has ever stuck with organized sports long enough to see how good they really could be. As a baseball player I had pretty good skills, but I was always undersized and really lacked the work effort to keep my small body in shape. Also, we never had the proper facilities in East Cleveland for me to train, even if I had wanted.

But Calvin has the body, the facilities, and the coaching. One fall Friday night in 1986, Natalie and I drive over to Lakewood to see Cleveland Heights play against powerful St. Ignatius High School. I can't believe my eyes when Calvin, wearing No. 97, goes around the left end and crashes into the quarterback for a sack. He looks so humongous on the field, not like my little cousin at all. In his junior year, his season is so successful that the coaches name him to the All-Lake Erie League team.

After so many years of wanting to see a real success story in my family, I really feel God is watching over Calvin and me. I am finally appreciating the value of a good education. And who knows? Calvin might be headed for college on a Division I football scholarship.

Others in our family are just as incredulous at Calvin's progression. He is spending regular hours in the weight room and beefing up so solidly that his mother, Pat, begins to question whether he is taking something to supplement his conditioning.

You're getting real big, Calvin, Pat tells him one afternoon at home. You're getting too big.

What you talking about, Ma? Calvin says.

Look, Pat says. You've seen I've fucked my life up with dope. I hope you aren't doing steroids. It's dope. That's all it is.

Calvin can't believe what he is hearing.

Mama, I ain't doing no steroids.

I'm gonna ask yo doctor if there's any in your blood system, she threatens.

Go right ahead, Calvin tells her.

Pat pushes the issue further, telling Big Calvin that he should check and make sure the team's coaches aren't giving the kids anything to make them bigger, stronger, faster.

Several weeks later, Big Calvin tells Pat that he's had a conversation with the team's head coach, and the coach assures him that no one is taking any performance-enhancing drugs to his knowledge.

Little Calvin continues to work out, waiting for the start of summer practice drills.

◪

Drills start in July, and they are grueling, made worse daily by the hot Cleveland sun. The team has two-a-days, which requires players to practice early in the morning and early in the evening.

Calvin is shining in practice, and the coaches are convinced he is going to be a real force when games start in September. In practice, he is hustling on each play, running out each wind sprint, and never skipping a single pushup. He is showing his teammates what leadership is all about.

After one particularly tough practice, Calvin and his best friend, Daryl, a Heights basketball player, hit a movie. When Calvin arrives home that night, he follows the voices he hears upstairs. His stepmother, Dana, and Michelle, his half sister, are sitting on a bed chatting. Michelle is laughing about something as Calvin walks in. Almost as soon as he goes to sit down, she stops and stares at him curiously.

Dag, Calvin, she says. What's wrong with your ankles?

He looks down. His right ankle is fat with swelling. Musta sprained it during practice today, he mumbles.

Uh-uh, Michelle says. That's not it. Both of them are swollen.

Dana takes a look. Calvin assures her that his ankles feel fine, and stepmom and son agree that he is probably just practicing too hard. He wants a scholarship to a Division I university. Calvin goes to bed. The ankle swelling is no big deal, he thinks.

Until the next morning, that is. The swelling is worse.

Bad enough that when Dana pokes an ankle, it leaves a fingerprint. Calvin and Dana head for the emergency room at University Hospitals of Cleveland. The doctors take blood and urine tests. After about an hour, a physician comes out to see them.

I have some news for the two of you, he says, as Calvin and Dana straighten up in their seats.

Calvin, the filters in your kidneys are putting out protein, and the protein is going into your body, the doctor says, getting to the point in a roundabout way. Normally, he explains, the protein would leave the body in the urine.

The doctor talks about something evil-sounding and complex called glomerulo nephritis sclerosis.

You have a kidney disease, Calvin, he says.

That, then, is the point.

Calvin and Dana sit silently, somberly. The doctor says the condition can be reversed with medication, and Calvin hears him talk about dialysis, a word he doesn't understand, and how it fortunately wouldn't be required. That means Calvin doesn't care about it.

The prescription: prednisone for the disease, and water pills to reduce the swelling. Once the swelling subsides, the doctor says, Calvin can resume football.

Calvin follows the doctor's orders and takes the medication regularly—until late August, a week before the season is to start. Heights High is to open its schedule against St. Joseph's, the school with Desmond Howard and some more highly touted players. Calvin, after several weeks on the prednisone, is feeling good, back to normal. His ankles aren't swelling. He feels as well as he ever has. He wants to do well in that first game. The college scouts will be on hand. He stops taking the prednisone.

He doesn't tell Big Calvin or Dana. He doesn't tell the

coaches. He doesn't even tell Daryl, his best friend.

Four days later, Dana goes to Calvin's room to see why he hasn't gotten up for football practice. She shakes him.

He is barely breathing.

He is foaming at the mouth.

◨

A siren cuts through the morning quiet on Goodnor Avenue in Cleveland Heights. Calvin is wheeled from his home and jammed into the back of the ambulance. The high school football star, felled and helpless, is on his way to the ER for the second time in a month.

For his decision to stop taking his kidney medicine, his body has repaid him with a blood clot in the lung. The doctors say they can treat the clot with Coumadin, a blood thinner. Blood thinners, of course, preclude contact sports. That means no more football, about as crushing a blow as Calvin has ever taken. That means his shot at a college scholarship has evaporated, for no school wants to hand out one of its precious rides to a kid who is sick.

It also means Calvin no longer will get by on the starstruck privilege conferred upon athletes; for the first time in his life, he has to look to something other than sports as a way of making his mark.

Initially, Calvin is depressed. He blames himself—and rightly so, because he decided to quit taking the prednisone pills that could have cured him. He realizes that he probably still would have been a step too slow to play Division I college football, as well as he had played the game in high school. And pro? Maybe it had just been a pipe dream.

Calvin begins focusing on the positive: He has his life, and if he takes his medicine, his health should return.

His senior year will be one of better grades, a full social life, and time with his girlfriend.

◩

I am aware that Calvin has been diagnosed with a kidney problem, and I know that it's a serious ailment. But I also know he's young and strong and I have total faith God will help him overcome it, as long as he doesn't stop taking his medication again.

Anyway, I have my own worries. Now that my senior year in college has started, I have taken over as editor-in-chief, and am concerned with making the *Cauldron*, the student newspaper, a good product. I also need to earn fifty-two credit hours between now and next summer in order to graduate.

To compound matters, I have had to quit my paying job at the *Plain Dealer* to run the *Cauldron*, even though I have a wife and a kid. It doesn't take long for us to get behind in our bills. Natalie is working at a secretarial job, but she is earning only about $5.25 an hour. Our bill paying goes into triage mode. We pay our rent and car note first because we have to have a place to live and a way to get downtown to school and work. One day, we get a letter saying that our twenty-inch floor-model color television will be repossessed if we don't come up with two monthly payments, the amount we owe. That night after Dwayne Jr. goes to sleep, Natalie and I sit in front of the television, the screen turned off, and gnash our teeth over the financial mess we are in. We don't have any relatives who are not in dire straits themselves, so we are on our own.

Natalie begins to sob uncontrollably. Dwayne, she says, we can't let them take our television. Why are these things happening to us?

It isn't that Natalie is concerned about missing her favorite shows. It's the idea that we are trying to break a cycle of poverty, and we are failing at it. I have quit a job that allowed us to pay the bills so I could get an education and some experience running a small paper. We believe those are the right moves, but now we are being punished for them.

For the rest of that week, Natalie works the phones trying to arrange payment of the television bill. She eventually lines up a loan and we pay it off, but now we have a loan-company bill with high interest rates we can't afford. The cycle is vicious.

All I want to do is finish college and get a real job to support this very real family I have made.

◪

I soon learn that my family is about to get bigger. Natalie finds out she is pregnant again. It's the summer of 1987 now, and I tell her we can't afford a second child. We are struggling badly enough, I have quit my job, and a new baby will put us under.

I have never much considered the abortion issue but I suggest we consider it. Natalie cries. She doesn't want to abort our child, but she knows I'm right about our economic situation. A baby means Natalie will have to quit working because her job is part time and she has no benefits. I have no benefits either. In order to bring this baby into the world, we will have to purchase medical insurance we can't afford.

We visit the office of Dr. Quentin Kenoyer, Natalie's physician. Natalie is still in her first trimester but she's not far from the second one. We need a decision now, because to wait any longer would be to lose the abortion option. Doctors are less apt to perform abortions after the first trimester, I have been told.

Finally, the nurse calls Natalie. She goes back for her consultation with the doctor, and I sit in the crowded waiting room reading a magazine. After about fifteen minutes, Natalie appears and says the doctor wants to see the two of us.

I go back and take a seat in the examination room. Natalie sits on the bed. Kenoyer is a thin, elderly doctor with glasses and gray in his hair. He has a soft-spoken, kind demeanor, almost timid. He makes some small talk before getting to the point. We need his referral before Natalie can get an appointment at the abortion clinic.

Kenoyer puts his hand on my shoulder and says he will not give us the referral. He says he's fundamentally opposed to abortion. He tells me about God and the preciousness of babies and how they are treasures and gifts.

Dwayne, he says, I have never made a referral for an abortion, even though many people have made that request. I've talked dozens of people out of making such a mistake. And you know what? Not one couple has regretted taking my advice years later, when they have seen their beautiful child grow and become part of their family.

I am angry with Quentin Kenoyer. Here he is complicating my already overwhelmed life. Who is he to tell us what to do? Is he going to pay our bills? Is he going to help me finish my education?

As much as I love Dwayne Jr., I can't afford another kid, financially or emotionally. Or can I? I think about how Grandma has always found a way, year after year. I realize—I hope—that she has taught me well.

Eventually I settle down and on January 6, 1988, our daughter is born. I named our son after me. Natalie gets to name our daughter. She chooses Christian Laine

Bray, although I think Christian is a boy's name. Natalie convinces me the name is gender-neutral.

◪

Other than our financial problems, my senior year at Cleveland State goes well. For the first time since I entered college, I am not working a regular job in addition to attending classes. I spend all day on campus, editing the paper and trying to make up for the credit hours I have blown off the previous four years. Under my leadership, the *Cauldron* does some hard-hitting stories and wins two major national college-newspaper awards, which is a coup considering Cleveland State only has a communication department and not a journalism school.

Around campus, I don't seem too popular with school authorities, especially Walter Waetjen, the university president. Waetjen and I start the academic year with a good relationship. He takes me to the private Cleveland Athletic Club for lunch. The only other blacks at the restaurant are busboys. Waetjen and I talk about the direction of the university and the direction of the news-paper under my stewardship. It is clear that he is trying to make sure we use the newspaper as just an extracur-ricular activity—not as a training ground for a future career in journalism. I respect his office but have no intentions of following his advice.

By February 1988, my relationship with Waetjen has soured. I see him at several university functions, but he either doesn't see me—which is hard because I am often the only black in attendance—or he chooses to ignore me.

The president is angry that I have allowed one of our columnists, Mark Lantz, to write scathing pieces that portray Waetjen as essentially a fool. Waetjen is partly right. Lantz can be extremely witty and brutal with his pen, and I probably should exercise more control over his column. After all, I am now the editor.

On the other hand, Lantz's work makes our paper lively. It is a local column on local university issues, and it is better than any column in the *Plain Dealer*. I often go around saying that if I ever become an editor at a daily newspaper, I will find Mark Lantz and instantly make him one of my columnists.

Mark's feature writing turns out to be the winner of one of our two national awards from the Gold Circle competition presented by the prestigious Columbia School of Journalism. The other award goes to me for my coverage of the university's basketball team. The team has had a three-year run in which it has gone to the NCAA Tournament and the NIT Tournament, has had a player die after a sudden heart ailment, and has been put on probation for recruiting Manute Bol, a seven-foot-six African who will wind up playing in the NBA.

My experience with Waetjen is invaluable. He is only the first of many prominent public officials who stop talking to me.

◫

It's winter 1988, and I am on schedule to graduate with the completion of one summer class. I set my sights on a summer internship with the *Plain Dealer*. I figure I have a shot. Their managing editor told me three years back to go to work for the *Cauldron* if I were serious about working in the industry. Not only have I joined the *Cauldron*, but I am editor-in-chief. My grades are only slightly above average, but I'm a hometown kid who, despite getting off track as a teen, has become a serious student of journalism. All of this has to impress the editors at the *Plain Dealer*, I'm sure.

I apply for the *Plain Dealer*'s internship program and land an interview for February 10, 1988, the morning my family is burying Grandma's sister, Aunt Dorothy (we always called her Aunt Red). She died at age fifty-nine of heart trouble.

Several days before the funeral, I tell Grandma I won't be there to pay my respects to Aunt Red. I say, This is an important interview I have. If they give me this job, it will help in the future because this is one of the best internships in the country. This is a good chance for me.

Honey, Red knows you love her, and we all gone be prayin' for you. We know that one day God gonna let you be the best news reporta there is. I knew that way back when those welfare people was talkin' about givin' my baby away. I said, I ain't givin' my own blood away. I told 'em, the Lord gone take care of us. And he is, too, child. So you gone on that interview. We'll bury Red.

It is a mild winter day when I leave my apartment in Warrensville Heights and catch three buses to downtown Cleveland to the *Plain Dealer* offices. My car is broken and Natalie and I don't have the money to get it fixed. But I'm not going to let a funeral or a broken-down car stop me from this big appointment.

I haven't walked through the double glass doors of the *Plain Dealer* on Superior Avenue since I left the circulation department six months earlier to become editor of the *Cauldron*. My interview is with an assistant editor. On my way up to the second-floor newsroom, I pass a couple of my old coworkers from the circulation department. We exchange pleasantries and I head to the interview.

The assistant editor is a relatively young guy, maybe in his early thirties. He looks like he needs some sleep and keeps rubbing his tired, bloodshot eyes. He asks me a few basic questions and, after about ten minutes, says thanks for coming, they'll let me know the outcome. I feel like I've been cheated. I wanted a real interview in which I would meet a series of editors and each would ask me probing questions about the stories I have written for the student newspaper. It is clear that this interview is super-ficial. If I ever become an editor, I promise myself, I will treat aspiring journalists with more respect.

It only takes a couple weeks for the rejection letter from the *Plain Dealer* to arrive. I try to turn my anger into something positive. But I can't forget that I am the newspaper editor of the college at Eighteenth and Euclid Avenue, and I applied for an internship at the daily news-paper at Eighteenth and Superior Avenue, just a couple blocks over, and they don't even give me a serious look. I begin to think, Where has all the effort I've put in the past couple years gotten me? Back to square one.

Then and there, I vow to hone my skills, to leave the streets behind forever, and to one day become a success so I can let my hometown newspaper know how much of a mistake it has made. Deep down, I know the *Plain Dealer* isn't at fault. They are big and can be discrimina-tory about whom their editors bring aboard. But I figure if I hold this against them it will make me more hungry and competitive.

I begin by applying to two other local newspapers. The *Lake County News Herald* in Willoughby, east of Cleveland, has a summer internship program. I apply and they invite me out for an interview. I had spent a day with some of their editors and reporters several years back as part of a classroom assignment at Cleveland State. These same editors tell me they believe I would be a good intern but that they are looking for someone who isn't so close to graduation. Lake County is mostly white, and I can't help but feel that my race is the reason they do not hire me. These thoughts scare me because I don't normally blame race for my rejections.

I also apply to the most respected paper in Ohio: the *Akron Beacon Journal*. At least this is painless. The editors in Akron don't even bother answering my query letter.

I am desperate. I'm no longer a kid. I'm a twenty-three-year-old man with a wife, two kids, and no job. I can go back to the *Plain Dealer* and beg for my circulation department job, or I can continue trying to land a job as a newspaper writer. I start looking through the *Editor & Publisher* yearbook for other newspapers in northeastern Ohio that might hire me. I figure if I am to land any job at a daily paper, it's going to be in a small newsroom that pays next to nothing.

❏

Poochie's father, Ted, manages a bar in a commercial district in East Cleveland. The area is dangerous, with several people having turned up murdered in the parking lot behind the place. Still, Poochie and I go there all the time, park in that murderous parking lot, and practically dare any of the gun-toting thugs to mess with us.

I am so used to hanging out that I am again losing any focus I have. But there always seems to be something that brings me back to reality. Poochie and I are in the bar one night, and his father's best friend, Skip, is finishing a drink. I sidle over and sit next to Skip. We talk and he remembers my mother and asks about her. I tell him she's in prison in Texas. She is hooked on drugs and keeps going in and out of the Texas Department of Corrections. Skip asks what I'm doing.

I'm going to Cleveland State, I say. I want to be a newspaper reporter. I have been doing some good stories at the student paper.

My nephew is into journalism, Skip says.

I straighten up immediately, drop my tough-man role. What you say? I ask Skip.

He works for the *Dayton Daily News*, Skip says. He's a reporter.

What's his name?

Mizell Stewart.

I had never heard this name before but I probe Skip for more information. Skip tells me that his cousin is my age and is even from Cleveland like me. I tell the bartender to take away my rum and Coke and bring me some coffee. My competitive juices start to flow. How could this Mizell person be my age, from my hometown, and already working at a big paper while I'm still trying to make it out of college?

I cross-examine Skip until early in the morning. I want to find out as much about Mizell as I can. If Mizell can make it, I figure, there's hope for me too.

◩

I stumble across information on the *Medina Gazette* in Medina County, about thirty-five miles southwest of Cleveland. It's within an hour's driving distance of Cleveland. The *Gazette*'s circulation is about seventeen thousand daily, which means it probably has two sportswriters. I send the editors my clips, but I am secretly hoping for rejection. The Lake County experience is still fresh in my mind, and I don't know if I want to go somewhere like Medina County, where the black population is almost nonexistent. In fact, from what I have heard in East Cleveland, there aren't any blacks in Medina County.

In the spring of 1988, I am sitting in my office at the student newspaper, somewhat distraught over the usual bills my wife and I can't pay. I am close to graduation and still don't have any real job prospect. I am wondering why I gave up my job and steady pay as a circulation clerk for this life of uncertainty. I had taken a gamble that newspapers would open their arms to me just because I am editor of the student newspaper and it turns out not to be true. But why is that? The paper continues to improve under my leadership, winning those two national awards, and pissing off the university president. Isn't that what journalism is all about? Throwing caution to the wind?

As I'm pondering these things, I get an unexpected call from Bob Hughes, the powerful chairman of the Republican Party in Cuyahoga County.

It is election time, and the biggest office in the land— the U.S. presidency—is up for grabs. But why is Hughes calling me? I've seen him on television and read about him in the papers, but he doesn't know me from any other college student.

Hughes quickly explains the nature of his call. He says that the Republican presidential nominee, Vice President George Bush, wants to come to Cleveland State and address the student body. University policy prohibits Waetjen or school officials from inviting Bush to campus because he is a partisan politician, just like his opponents Jesse Jackson and Michael Dukakis. Hughes explains that, as the head of a student organization, I have the authority to invite Bush to campus as a speaker. And if I will use this power to extend the vice president an invitation, the Republican Party will do me a huge favor.

For a moment, I wonder if they will pay all my bills, fix my car, buy clothes for my children. But that's not the offer.

We will get you an interview with the vice president, Hughes says.

You mean I will talk one-on-one with George Bush? I ask.

That's right, Hughes said. Bush wants to get closer to the people. He isn't giving interviews to the *Plain Dealer* or any of the big papers, just your student paper.

Mr. Hughes, if you can keep your promise, you've got a deal, I said.

I hang up the phone and thrust a sheet of paper into my Hendrix typewriter. I address it to the Office of the Vice President of the United States and invite him to Cleveland State. I realize that Bush is a Republican who has defended some of President Ronald Reagan's conservative policies. This will leave my invitation up for criticism because Cuyahoga County is a Democratic stronghold. After talking to Gary Engle, an English professor and the advisor of the student newspaper, I decide to send letters of invitation to both Dukakis and Jackson. Of course neither of them will respond, but at least I cover my butt. I also write an editorial in the paper explaining that as a newspaper editor, I want to bring all three presidential candidates to campus to open a dialogue on important issues in this country and our student body. The strategy works in that no one criticizes me too harshly for inviting the Republican Bush to campus.

◩

George Bush is on his way to Cleveland State and, as usual, I am running late for our meeting. Instead of getting a good night's sleep, I was hanging around with Poochie, telling him about my big interview. Now I am paying for it. I am supposed to be at Cleveland State in a conference room waiting for Bush two hours before his speech, but it is ninety minutes before speech time and I am just pulling into the university parking lot.

I get out of my car and there pulling up next to me is another vehicle. Out of it steps Don King, the boxing promoter. He ignores me. He is with a very tall, attractive woman. I figure she is probably his spokeswoman. She looks like one of those women who walks around the boxing ring between rounds holding up the cards.

I find the door I'm supposed to enter and someone with Bush's party—he may be a Secret Service guy—tells me I'm late and that I might not be able to talk with the vice president because they usually don't let anyone in this late due to safety concerns. Finally, after talking with someone on a walkie-talkie, he opens the door and I am allowed in, as thousands of Bush supporters (and some protesters) remain outside the building in a carnival-like atmosphere. I walk into a lower-level conference room and the vice president's staff and many Secret Service agents are ringed around the room. At a table in the center are two journalists, Jonathan Riskind of the *Lake County News Herald* and someone from the *Lorain Journal*. So much for my one-on-one interview with the vice president. Hughes hadn't been exactly honest with me.

Finally, after about an hour's wait, George Bush strides to the table and introduces himself, as if he needs an introduction. He says hi to the other reporters, the professional ones. When he is introduced to me, Bush says, Dwayne, nice to meet you. And thanks for inviting me to Cleveland State.

Oh, he is so good, I am thinking.

Here is the vice president, and he takes time out to thank me, personally. The interview lasts fifteen minutes too long, and Bush's staff is antsy, looking at their watches and talking into their portable radios. The staffers try to rush him, but he tells them he wants to answer all of our questions.

After the interview, as Bush is preparing to address the several thousand supporters, I walk out of the conference room with him and he asks me what year I am. He wants to know my plans after college and how long I've been with the student paper. I am impressed. I like the man, if not his politics. I devote two full pages in the next edition of the *Cauldron* to the interview.

◩

It's June 1988, and I am just getting home after a long day on campus. The phone rings and the guy on the other end identifies himself as Harlan Spector, city editor of the *Medina Gazette*. We talk for a while and he invites me to Medina for an interview. Oh boy, I'm thinking, what have I gotten myself into? The prospect of working at a place where I might be the only black is frightening. But what other coals do I have in the fire?

I drive down Interstate 71, exit at State Route 18, go past miles of undeveloped land and into the beautiful city of Medina, which is the county seat. Medina is quaint and home to nineteen thousand residents. The centerpiece of the city is a restored, picture-perfect downtown where streets are lined with late, nineteenth-century-style electric lights. Set in the middle of downtown is a Victorian public square, with a gazebo and bandstand, the perfect place for townsfolk to get together for ice-cream socials, summer concerts, and political speeches. Overlooking the square from the east is a mid-nineteenth-century courthouse with a pair of projecting wings, prominent quoins, a two-story recessed portico, and a mansard roof with a projecting tower clock. On the west side of this gorgeous square are eleven two- and three-story brick storefronts, including the trendy Main Street Café, that bustles with traffic from lunch to closing time. So beautiful is this downtown that NBC has dubbed Medina "Hometown, USA." I feel like I am driving through a fairy tale.

◩

Harlan is in his early thirties. He is about five foot eight and has a receding hairline. He is very calm and soft-spoken, and offers me a drink. Harlan introduces me to Liz Schaefer, the managing editor, who smiles and laughs easily. Both editors are very cordial. He has told me over the phone that no sports writing or cityside reporting jobs are open, but we discuss a position as a business reporter. I feel this county and this job prospect are both out of my range.

A few days later, Harlan calls and offers me the job. He says the pay is not much, $220 a week. When I call back to decline, based on pay, Harlan says give him a few days, maybe he can do something about the pay. He seems to like me.

I'm hoping he can't work any magic to change the pay

offer. I don't want to work in Medina County, and I don't want to earn $220 a week. I was earning $270 a week as a part-time customer service rep at the *Plain Dealer.* Now I'm being asked to take fifty dollars less a week to be a full-time reporter with a college degree?

Harlan calls back and says, I can offer you $230 a week, plus benefits.

I want to say no, but I'm liking this Harlan guy more and more. And since I have two small kids, the benefits will come in handy.

I take the job, with great reservations. I only know the inner city and downtown Cleveland. I am moving out of my comfort zone, and this is scary business. Would Harlan move out of his comfort zone to take a job in the inner city like East Cleveland? No. So why am I doing it?

◧

Being a business reporter in Medina County isn't so tough or bad. They usually work me four or five overtime hours a week, so that gets my pay up an extra thirty dollars or so. Plus, the work involves mostly writing soft business features. Five months into the job, I am promoted to the Brunswick City Hall beat. Brunswick, a bedroom community of about thirty thousand people, is the county's largest city. It is mostly blue-collar and many of the residents work in or around Cleveland, having moved to Brunswick to escape the ills of big-city life. On Friday nights, sports editor Bob Finan usually asks me to help his staff cover football or basketball games, which I am more than happy to do because it provides me with some deadline sports writing and it gives me more much-needed overtime.

Doug Oster and I are riding along a rural road looking for a Medina County woman who is accused of bilking a company out of hundreds of thousands of dollars. Doug is the chief photographer for the *Gazette*. I don't know him or anyone else in Medina well. I've only been on the job a couple of months.

We are making small talk when Doug says something that catches my attention.

I bet people out here have a lot to talk about when you leave their offices, Doug says.

I laugh softly and say, What's that supposed to mean?

Well, you've gotta be one of the first black reporters they've come across, he says.

Doug isn't trying to offend. He is a brilliant shooter, but like most photographers I've met, he is better with pictures than with words. When he talks, his thoughts come out raw and without nuance. But he is a nice guy. The fact is, he is mouthing what is on the minds of many others. Doug is trying to gauge how I feel about being the only black reporter in the county—maybe the first ever. But I decide not to give him any insights. I want my work to do all the talking.

My reaction makes me feel good. In earlier years, I would have challenged Doug, asked him why he felt compelled to put me on the spot. But now I am learning to handle adverse situations without always having to rely on the defense mechanism of fighting back. It feels good, this new sense of security in myself.

Several months after that conversation I am near the main square in the center of Medina. I am low on gas and out of cash. I see a cash machine and head for it. A white woman in her early thirties has just pulled out her ATM card. She is about to stick it in the machine but turns around quickly. She is panicking, as if I'm about to rob her. I stand behind the imaginary line, waiting for my turn. The woman, however, is trembling. If a cop were nearby, I am convinced she would call him and tell him I am trying to rob her.

Even in my most decadent times, I never would have robbed anyone. I've come so far, yet my progress makes no difference to some of the whites of Medina County, many of whom moved here—far away from Cleveland and its ghettos—to get away from people who look like me. I don't think these people hate blacks, but they know years of oppression, from yesterday's slavery to today's subpar public schools, have led to a second-class existence for blacks in the United States. And these whites don't want to have to face that every day. But my mere presence reminds them of what it is they are fleeing. And now I understand why blacks, even black professionals, never find peace in suburbia. Because to some whites, blacks will always be suspicious. Suspected of something.

The woman at the ATM turns, still shaking, and looks at me.

Sir, she says, why don't you use the machine before me?

I snicker. I have to get to Brunswick for a meeting with Skip Trimble, the longtime city manager. I don't have time to be angry. I am amused. I do as the woman says. Then I go and interview Skip about his lengthy tenure as city manager. When I leave his office, I ask myself what he thinks of me. What if Doug is right?

I am convinced that Skip, the man who runs the largest city in Medina County, just sees me as a reporter, not as a black guy who one day might rob him.

In Medina, I learn that I have a gift for reporting daily newspaper stories. I also learn that I have a lot to learn if I want to become a strong writer. Harlan works to patch up holes in my story. He has been at the paper for nearly a decade and knows the ins and outs of the county better than most people in the newsroom.

Liz and Harlan both seem to believe I have a future in the business, and their faith gives me the confidence to take some chances in my reporting. But clearly there are reporters at the *Gazette* who are more seasoned than I. Rob Whitehouse, the courts reporter, is young and handsome and smart. Very smart. His girlfriend, Tammy Lash, might be smarter than Rob. She is ambitious, too, and clearly wants to move on to bigger and better things. Tammy and Rob are a great couple. To acclimate myself to the county, I read a series of stories she has done on blacks here. She reports that the county is less than 1 percent black and that most of them live in an isolated area in Medina.

Most of our staff on the news side of things are in their twenties. Ron Coulter, the Medina city beat reporter, is someone I can talk to because, like me, he is a young husband and father. He is also a sharp guy with a dry wit. Ron seems to be more worldly than many of the others. While most of these reporters are about my age, they haven't spent the last eight, nine years hanging out on rough innercity streets, refusing to study, and some days being lucky just to stay out of jail, prison, or the graveyard.

That's probably why I decide that whatever problems I had in the past are behind me, and that from this day on I will try to outhustle everyone on every reporting assignment I get. I don't want to appear too aggressive or ambitious, but I want to compete. I figure competition will help keep me focused on my goal of one day getting a job at a larger newspaper.

◪

I am sitting at my desk chatting with a colleague, when a coincidence of cosmic proportions unfolds. My phone rings, and on the other line is none other than Mizell Stewart. I have spent hours talking about Mizell with his uncle Skip, my cousin Ted's friend. I have never met Mizell, never even talked to him, but he is the guy who has been living out my dream of working for a large daily newspaper, writing about everyday life in the city. I have admired his success, based on what Skip has told me, and now to my astonishment, here he is on my phone line.

We are the same age, but Mizell is so far ahead of me in his career that I give him the courtesy of someone who is much older, much more experienced. I'm not sure he notices how in awe of him I am. I am twenty-four, and so is he. But when he asks a question, I say, Yes, sir and no, sir. He laughs and says to just call him Mizell. What a guy!

Mizell says he's heard I am a promising young reporter. The *Dayton Daily News* has an opening in its neighborhood news section and might be interested in talking to me about the job. He wants to know if I'd be interested. Of course, I tell him. He says he'll let his editor know about me. A few days later, one of Mizell's editors calls. Ron Rollins offers me a formal interview.

I tell Harlan, and he just says, I figured a bigger paper would come after you sooner or later.

I'm confused by his comment. Everybody in our newsroom wants to go to a bigger paper, even Harlan. He has been at the *Gazette* about nine years but has had no luck moving up. I've only been here one year and now one of the nation's top sixty newspapers is banging on my door. Is Harlan suggesting that bigger newspapers would give me a shot before my time because they need black reporters to cover the increasingly black inner cities? It confuses me because I think Rob Whitehouse, in particular, is much more talented than I am. Why has the Dayton paper called me and not Rob? His skills are several years ahead of mine.

I conclude that Harlan is trying to pay me a compliment, not take a shot at me. He thinks I'm a good reporter, hard working. But the reality is also that newspapers, once the bastion of white males, are also trying to better integrate their staffs. So when they look at two promising young reporters like Rob and myself, most editors are starting to give the nod to the black reporter.

I am putting way too much thought into the implications of my job interview in Dayton. Anyway, Rob is a single guy without a wife and kids. I am married and can barely meet my financial obligations working at a small newspaper.

My interview will last two days, even though I've only brought one suit—my only suit, a brown, tweed number that is getting to be a little tight almost everywhere. Ron told me I'd be here for one day only. Steve Sidlo, the managing editor, grills me over lunch with a lot of hypothetical questions. If I'm covering city hall and find out that the mayor has recommended giving a contract to a client from his law firm, how would I pursue the story? We are at lunch: Sidlo, Ron, and metro editor Jim Ripley. I am trying to eat, but every time I dig my fork into the bass and pasta on my plate, out flies another question from this hard-nosed trio. The food is flying off their plates and into their bellies. They are full and still asking questions. My food goes nowhere because they won't give me a chance to eat.

Finally on my second day in Dayton, in the same suit I wore the first day, it is time to visit with the most important person in the newsroom: Max Jennings, the editor.

Max, an excitable type with a strong reputation of defending the First Amendment, has a thick mane of black hair graying at the sides. He looks at you and smiles and gives the impression that he knows more than others. He doesn't like me, that's clear off the bat. Max grills me about a whole variety of issues and says he doesn't believe I can cut it in Dayton. I sit across from this important man in his large, fifth-floor corner office and feel like I'm drowning. I need air but he doesn't give me any. In fact, he takes away what oxygen I have remaining.

Why does a guy like yourself think you can leave a small suburban paper to come here to the big time? he asks.

I am not prepared for this. I tell him that stories in Dayton are no different from stories in Medina. You report and write them the same way. He is not impressed and later tells the managing editor and the metro editor not to hire me.

To my surprise, Sidlo and Ripley fight their boss on the issue. Dwayne has potential, they say. Sure, he's a little unrefined but that's OK. And then they hit him with their best punch: We owe it to our readers to diversify, to bring on young minorities and help them grow. It can only help readership if we have a staff that's more reflective of the community. We only have a couple black male reporters out of a staff of about seventy. We need to give this kid a chance. And we need to give him a good, somewhat high-profile beat assignment. We need to have him cover the Dayton Police Department.

I had told them how I grew up in the inner city. I had told them I think I'm a tough reporter because of my background. Now they are using the same argument with their boss. Max relents and goes to publisher Brad Tillson for the okay to hire me at a starting salary of $585 a week. Tillson signs off. After all this is worked out behind closed doors, Ripley comes down to the newsroom and finds me. I am sitting at the metro desk, marveling at the crackle of all the various police scanners and the activities. I am frightened by all the action. Then Ripley offers me the job. I accept but feel I am getting in over my head. I am afraid that Max is right.

◩

Before leaving for Dayton, Natalie and I spend two weeks wrapping up our affairs in Cleveland. Our families are proud of us. We seem to be the only ones who have a real chance of breaking the cycle of poverty that has been so prevalent in our families for generations. I spend a lot of time hanging out on Brightwood, drinking with old friends. One of them is David Alexander, the uncle of one of my childhood friends. He has just returned from California after going out there almost a decade earlier. David, my uncles Antmo and Bill, and I sit around almost every evening drinking beer and telling lies, waiting for me to head off to Dayton.

David has some severe leg injuries that cause him to walk with a bad limp. He doesn't talk about them much, but Bill says some gang members tied him to a car and dragged him through the streets of South-Central Los Angeles. Dave says he had been part of a notorious gang and mentions murder and other things in which he had been involved. Another lie, I say one day, and tell him to just hand me a cold beer. We laugh and change the subject every time Dave talks about his gang life, driving a 5.0 Mustang one hundred miles per hour and other such nonsense. California seems so distant, Dave's stories seem so made up.

A week after I leave for Dayton, I return with a front-page story I have written. Dave is the first guy I run across, and I pull out the paper and show him.

You've been down there just one week, he says, and you're already writing front-page stories. He gives me a high five. I stay the weekend and return to Dayton. My grandma calls one night and says the FBI has just raided our house on Brightwood.

That boy Dave Alexander apparently had killed somebody out in California, she says. The FBI had been watching him for a while, probably even when you were out there sitting with him. They thought Bill was part of that mess or something. They came up the street in these U-Haul trucks, and we all thought somebody was moving. But they jumped out of the back with these big old guns, and they ran over to Mr. Alexander's house and kicked in the door and went in and were looking for David.

Another whole truck full of them ran over to my house and came right in with guns and pointed them at my head, Grandma says. They were looking for yo Uncle Bill, boy.

I put it together: Dave hadn't been lying about his gang activity and the murders. Word is that he was on the FBI's Most Wanted list. That he planned a murder, went to the wrong house, and killed an innocent man.

I know Dave as the All African-American boy across the street. Light-skinned, tall, a former guard on the Shaw High School basketball team. His dad, a widower, raised a large family on Brightwood, worked hard, kept a clean, neat yard. I admired Dave for being an athlete and for being conversant in many different topics, from sports to politics to geography. By the time I meet up with him in the late 1980s, I'm college educated and embarking on a career in journalism. And Dave's leg is mangled, a result of his violent lifestyle. He is on the lam, unbeknownst to me. Hanging around with Dave for a few summer months, I never realize how close I am to being hauled off to jail or worse—being gunned down. It is just one of many chances a ghetto boy like myself takes by merely getting up in the morning and doing nothing at all.

◩

In September 1989, Calvin is enrolled in his second year of classes at Akron University. To help make ends meet, he begins driving a postal truck in Copley Township outside Akron. During the first week of his sophomore year, he feels flu-ish and weak. At Akron General Hospital, just like at University Hospitals three years earlier, the lab work again tells the tale: Calvin's kidneys have given out. Extremely high blood pressure, a doctor says. Stroke risk.

You need dialysis to stay alive, the doctor says. In other words, Calvin will have to have all the blood taken from his body and run through a machine to cleanse it. The procedure will leave him feeling spent. And the doctor tells him he needs to have these treatments three times a week or he will become sicker and probably die.

Little Calvin is alone, devastated. He phones Big Calvin, sobbing.

Daddy, he says. It came back.

What came back? his father says.

My kidney problems came back.

By the time Big Calvin and other relatives make the forty-five-minute drive from Cleveland to Akron, Calvin is already hooked up to the dialysis machine. A shunt is implanted in his chest to provide the connection to his body through which the mechanical kidneys can do their work.

Calvin is told that the only way he can escape these procedures and still live is by having a kidney transplant.

◻

Other relatives keep me abreast of Calvin's medical problems, but by now I am 225 miles away. I love my cousin, but being away from home seems to make it easier for me to rely on others to help him.

In Dayton, James E. Newby becomes the most important man in my daily life. Newby is Dayton's chief of police. A longtime street officer and sergeant with strong ties to the police union, Newby talks with the small-town accent of his native Hillsboro, deep in southern Ohio. He usually has a rich tan even in the dead of winter, it appears. He is short, perhaps five foot eight, and reminds me of Napoleon because he talks tough and has a no-nonsense approach.

Why is it that the *Dayton Daily News* believes it can put a rookie reporter like you on the police beat all the time? Newby says to me during our first meeting.

I am offended by the question. But Newby is right: I'm inexperienced and probably over my head trying to report on the daily operations of a police department with nearly five hundred sworn officers.

No offense, Newby continues, but before you they had Phillip Morris on the beat.

Phil was even greener than me when he took over this job two years ago. He was fresh out of college. Now it's my turn, and I'm just a year out of college.

All I ask is that you be fair, Newby says.

With that, Napoleon dismisses me, and I leave, not knowing what to make of him.

◧

In Dayton, life improves somewhat for Natalie, the kids, and me. I am finally making some decent money. She gets a job as a secretary at a tool-and-die shop, which Dayton seems to have plenty of. She doesn't work long, however, because Dwayne Jr. has started to have large-scale seizures brought upon by fevers. Natalie theorizes that our son contracts colds and the flu from other kids in day care, so she decides to become a stay-at-home mom, which sinks us back into financial ruin.

That March in Cleveland, Big Calvin gives Little Calvin a kidney. He wants to do whatever he can to help out his son, including giving the young man a piece of him. But Big Calvin has led a rough life, one of constant ripping and running in the streets, heavy drinking, fighting, stints in jail. His body is worn down and the doctors know it. They don't want to go through with the operation. But Big Calvin is a persuasive man. He tells the doctors there is no way they are going to deny him the opportunity to save the life of his first-born son. Meanwhile, Little Calvin isn't doing well on dialysis; his blood is clotting all the time. So the doctors relent and perform the operation.

It isn't a total success. During the surgery, Big Calvin's lung is punctured, and we are afraid he is going to die. He pulls through after a stint in intensive care. Little

Calvin's new kidney certainly improves his health, but not as dramatically as had been hoped. He remains in the hospital for weeks and his creatinine, a waste product of the muscle that is taken care of by the kidneys, remains excessively high. His skin doesn't regain its full color and pimples pockmark his face.

But the kidney is good enough that, with all the medication, Little Calvin doesn't need dialysis anymore and that in and of itself is a partial victory. Within several months, Big Calvin and his son are both able to return to somewhat normal lives.

The doctors tell Little Calvin that he will be home free if the transplanted kidney survives three years.

With the job in Dayton, I know I have come a long way from my origins. I am college educated, a father and husband, and now an employee for one of the largest media companies in the United States. Several former *Dayton Daily News* staffers have gone on to work in the company's corporate offices while others have become some of the nation's top journalists.

I am not too worried about what the future might hold in mid-1990 because I know just handling the police beat in Dayton is a tough enough assignment. But I still have some very competitive juices, and I understand that any future success hinges on how I perform as a reporter in Dayton, Ohio.

No one ever puts pressure on me to succeed. My mother used to keep on me to perform well in school, but once she discovered drugs she lost interest. Grandma never expected me to do anything more than get married, get a job, and take care of my family. No one ever expected me to finish college and get a white-collar job. Nobody other than myself.

And I don't know where this drive came from. I only know that since I was a boy, I've always had a competitive streak. In my youth, it led me to try out for the baseball team year after year. It kicked in when I lived in Mississippi and competed with my classmates for the best grade in algebra, but in truth it didn't really take root in my intellectual life until I was older. And now it had shadowed me to Dayton.

The editors in Dayton seem to send me to every fire and police call that comes across the scanners. But I quickly realize that along with improving my writing, the main thing I have to do is come up with my own good stories. If you do that, the editors don't bother assigning you work they have dreamed up in a meeting. They let you go on your own, and call you a self-starter and give you nice raises.

While most of my competition, especially television reporters, waste time talking to each other at fire and crime scenes, I usually head off into the crowds and talk to neighbors and other onlookers. They are the ones who know the community best. I learn a lot this way about my new city, and I start to develop sources and my own story ideas.

I am most concerned with allegations I have read in the paper accusing certain Dayton police officers of brutality. In largely black West Dayton, residents give me horror stories about a pair of cops who allegedly call themselves Batman and Robin and use excessive force to get confessions and other information. I figure these claims are exaggerated. Many of these people have no jobs or income and make their living hustling in the streets. The highlight of their day can be showing up at a crime scene and trying to look important by talking to reporters. They especially like getting in front of the television cameras and pretending to know what's going on, all the while butchering the Queen's English. I find this amazing because back in East Cleveland I would never have gotten in front of a television camera at a crime scene because perpetrators know how to retaliate. Exaggerated or not, I am concerned about these allegations of misconduct, so I begin delving into internal affairs investigations.

◼

The police chief Newby doesn't like my style of reporting at all. Within my first year on the beat, I ink a series of stories that details these complaints of police misconduct. Newby is livid when I visit him in his office after the stories begin running. He wastes no time trashing me.

Let me tell you something, he says, shaking his head in disgust. Those stories you've been writin' in the paper are a piece of shit!

I sit facing him across his desk. It's like I am a student being scolded by the principal. I can't believe a big-city police chief is saying these things to me, but at least I know he's paying attention to what I'm writing.

You take a few complaints made against a few officers and you make a big deal about them, Newby says. What you have to realize is that those complaints were found to be unsustained, which means we don't know if the excessive force did happen or didn't happen, and if it did happen, we don't know if it was justified or not. Just because someone complains about a police officer doesn't make them right. Our officers have to go into all kinds of situations, dealing with drug addicts who don't want to go to jail, going into domestic-violence situations, and dealing with people who are stoned out of their minds.

He continues, I don't think you know what you're doing. You shouldn't write these kinds of articles until you know what you're doing.

Newby sets his steely eyes on me and says he can find only one thing redeeming in this whole affair—the fact that I didn't write the stories and then try to avoid him.

Not many people in this city are going to say something like that about me and my department and then have the guts to come into my office the next day and look me in the eye, he says.

Is he trying to praise me?

I can give you credit for that, Newby says.

I leave, standing by my stories, even though deep down I know they have some flaws and the chief isn't totally off base. Perhaps I am too new in town to be tackling such a weighty issue as police brutality. In my probe, I have found a lot of smoke but no fire. I have never found that one irrefutable clue, the so-called "smoking gun," that would make the case.

Although I would never tell the chief, I admire him in a way. He has been a street officer working the beat. He has been a sergeant, supervising in the trenches. And he now runs the department. He has a bachelor's and a master's degree. I always think how lucky I would be if my journalism career someday parallels Newby's police career. I decide that I want to get a master's degree at some point.

About eight months after the excessive-force stories are published, I get my big break. A detective stops me in the halls of the Dayton Safety Building and says, They are trying to fire John Gamble.

John Gamble is the only young black officer on the department's street-level undercover narcotics team. I don't know Gamble so I begin asking around about him, but most of my sources have no information about why he's being investigated by internal affairs.

I am sitting in the office one day later that same week and a thick pile of bound paper comes flying over my left shoulder and lands on my desk.

There's your proof, veteran reporter Wes Hills says.

Proof of what? I ask.

Of what they have been doing over at the Dayton Police Department for years, Hills says, a serious look on his face.

Hills, the paper's longtime federal courts reporter, has gotten his hands on a thick internal affairs report and the name on the cover catches my attention: John Gamble.

I take the report home and read it that night on my living room couch. It documents a six-month investigation into claims that Gamble and at least one other officer tortured a suspect with a scalding-hot clothes iron during a drug raid. The report says that Officer Ron Norton held the suspect down while Gamble applied the hot instrument to the suspect's body and threatened to burn off his genitals if the suspect didn't answer the officers' questions. A third officer, Terry Hunt, allegedly stood guard.

Our large headline runs over six columns the next day: Police Burn Man with Hot Iron.

I am immediately dispatched along with a photographer to the Southeastern Corrections Facility prison to interview defendant/victim David Greer. Greer is only nineteen and appears younger. He is skinny and shy, and treats me like I'm an authority, although I try to put him at ease by talking to him in the language of the streets. In Greer I literally see myself, lost on the streets all those years. The drug crack wasn't sold when I was a teen, but if it had been, I'm not sure I would have been able to escape being a prisoner to it.

When I arrive back in the newsroom, the place is electric. Nothing energizes a newsroom like a big story, and this is one. Newby is holding a press conference at city hall to announce that Gamble, Norton, and Hunt have been fired. Bob Siller, the special agent in charge of the FBI, announces that his agents are investigating the incident. Television and radio are abuzz with the story of the out-of-control Dayton cops.

I take no pleasure in this. I know that most of the cops in Dayton work hard and respect people's rights. I know all this attention is unfair because they put their lives in jeopardy each and every day. But at the same time, I know that Newby needs to exercise tighter control over the drug units.

Several months later the city of Dayton agrees to pay Greer $300,000 to drop his lawsuit. The FBI investigation leads to a guilty plea by Officer Norton to misdemeanor charges. Gamble is never convicted and is later shot and killed outside a West Dayton bar over a dispute with the bar's owner.

Throughout my tenure in Dayton, Newby suggests that I should report more on what's happening on the streets and less on what's going on in the police department. I feel, however, that I can have more of an impact on how the police department handles crime by making sure officers stay in line and have the proper staffing and equipment. But, as usual, the streets beckon. Only this time, I am not hustling—I'm a reporter.

◩

A young black man they call Sweetback races over to a red truck that slows to a stop on Piqua Place in Southern Dayton View. The truck pulls out of sight, into a cul-de-sac. Within seconds, a gunshot shatters the passenger-side window, leaving a hole as a big as a baseball. The truck speeds off.

Sweetback walks over to me. This is what Newby meant by covering the streets. Sweetback has a brownish snub-nosed .357 Magnum in his right hand. He opens the cylinder of the revolver, flicks away the spent brass casings and inserts a fresh cartridge. He looks me in the eye.

That motherfucka tried to drive off with my shit, he says, meaning his crack cocaine.

I'm standing in the middle of Summit Court, one of Dayton's most notorious havens for crack, violence and economic despair. At places like Summit Court, young black men compete for drug profits in a seemingly lawless environment ruled by intimidation. Brutal force has become so common around this housing project that the dealers refer to the neighborhood as "the Jungle."

I come here because another reporter and I are working on a series of stories called "License to Deal." The newspaper has used a computer to study the arrest patterns in Montgomery County and has concluded that Summit Court has had more drug arrests than any other neighborhood in the county. We interview probation officers, cops, judges, and jailed offenders and their families. Somehow, I get the bright idea that the series isn't complete unless we go out and hang around a drug hot spot and see for ourselves what's motivating young men to put their lives on the line to sell drugs. And of course, I would be the one to go out to do the reporting.

I am fortunate that Marlon Shackelford, a community activist, agrees to escort me over to Summit Court. I tried going there by myself once, but had a pistol pointed at me so I left.

Now it is early June 1992, and I am back. Marlon is blunt and, as we approach a group of young gun-toting toughs, he tells them I'm a reporter and says it's important that they give me the scoop on why they sell dope.

Marlon says, We don't want no names. We ain't the police. We just a couple young brothers just like all y'all. Just tell us why y'all sell dope. We're cool.

The dope dealers want none of this. Nobody around here sells no dope, says one. The man, who is twenty, puts his hand on a gun strapped to his waistband. That's why I got this, he says, brandishing the gun. To make sure nobody sells dope.

It's hard not to be edgy at Summit Court, and now I'm thinking Newby knew all this when he suggested that I cover the streets more, get out among the dope dealers and abusers.

After about an hour, the young men start to open up to me. Tutu walks over to Sweetback and some of the others. Tutu puts his arms around their shoulders. He says, This is how it is: we're black and we're held back because of our color. We don't wait on no white folks.

The men say they have no real hope of escaping the ghetto and—with no jobs or education—are living life the best way they know how. For now that means protecting their turf.

Everyone is standing between two tenements on Shawano Place, which sits off Piqua. Graffiti spray-painted on one of the beige brick buildings sums up the men's feelings: Fuck the Police.

The only time the police come down here is election time, Sweetback says. He smokes a joint and sits next to Marlon on some steps. Tutu hands his forty-ouncer of Crazy Horse beer to someone in the crowd and starts talking about guns. At night, he says, it's like Beirut around here.

We don't want to hurt nobody, Tutu tells me. We want to survive. But if you get in the way, you get stepped on.

◪

My day in the projects is action-packed. Sweetback pistol-whips a woman for buying crack from someone other than him. The cops cruise down and everyone—including me for some reason—runs into the bowels of the projects where we can't be caught. But perhaps the most tense moment comes after the cops take off. Someone yells, Those are dem boys from Cincinnati!

Several dealers pull their pistols. Everybody looks for cover. I don't know where to go. Just a few years ago, I was so hip to the ways of the streets, but now I act as if I don't know what to do when someone pulls a pistol.

The car they are talking about is coming in our direction. Pretty fast, too. I see that four or five young males are in it. I suspect more violence is on the way, may even be headed for me. The car gets closer. The dealers I have been talking to are ready for battle. A woman yells, Get my babies out the way!

I am confused about which way to turn. It seems that

I am the only one out in the open. And all I have for protection is a reporter's notebook.

Finally someone says, That's not them.

Just like that, peace is restored to Summit Court. And I get my story.

◪

That August Natalie, the kids, and I leave Dayton, where we have been for three years, because I have been accepted as a Kiplinger Fellow in the journalism program at Ohio State. By going back to school, I am putting my family further and further into debt. In Dayton I have a good job and am earning nearly forty thousand dollars a year. But my bad undergrad grades have been gnawing at me, and I want to obtain a master's degree to make up for them. My metro editor, Jim Ripley, tries to convince me that I don't need an advanced degree, but I am dead set on the move. At Ohio State, I am enrolled in a program for journalists with at least three years experience.

My undergraduate grades alone weren't good enough to get me into Ohio State, but the program professor tells me my reporting work on the Dayton Police Department worked in my favor during the selection process.

◪

Some people say their time as a Kiplinger Fellow at Ohio State is the most interesting year of their life. For me, it is a year in which I am determined to make amends for my sorry undergraduate performance and to learn as much as I can about the world in which I live. I am a student at Ohio State, a claim I have wanted since I saw Woody Hayes coach the Buckeye team in the Rose Bowl in 1969.

What the program offers me, though, is a window through which to view how rapidly my life is changing. I am in grad school and part of a class of eight professionals that has special status on this campus of more than fifty thousand students. People are starting to look up to me, call me a success. But I know better—I know that less than ten years earlier I was growing up on the streets, shooting dice, cutting school, and believing that I had blown any shot I had at making something of myself.

Except for that fact that I'm broke, the "Kip" year is fulfilling. My stipend for the year totals about $18,000, far less than what I earned in Dayton, but enough for us to survive because Natalie takes a part-time job as a store clerk. I take a full class load and earn As in every subject, except for a B in an English class.

The director of our program, Mike Masterson, is a former investigative reporter and editor from Arkansas who has many interesting connections. We focus a lot on the upcoming election and a candidate Mike knows from Arkansas named Bill Clinton. Mike predicts Clinton will win in November, which of course he does. Another of Mike's friends is talk-show host Geraldo Rivera, whom he recruits to come to Columbus and spend the day with us. Despite my negative opinions about Geraldo as a newsman, he is so down-to-earth in person that I end up liking the guy. Meeting celebrity newsmen, debating national politics—it's a stimulating time for me.

The school year goes by fast for all of us in the program, but especially for me: I land a job at the *Los Angeles Times* in the middle of the year. As a result, I need to finish the Kip program in ten months instead of eleven. I do so and take off, back to a working world where the pay is much better.

In the course of ten years, I have gone from selling hot dogs at ballgames in Cleveland to a job reporting for the *Los Angeles Times*, one of the five largest newspapers in the country. Southern California is expensive, but with overtime I am earning nearly sixty thousand dollars a year. We live in a coastal town called Ventura. Ventura County sits between Los Angeles and Santa Barbara Counties off Highway 101.

I can't believe how blessed I am. Natalie, the kids, and I frequently go to the Ventura harbor, where we sit on the restaurant-lined pier and eat calamari and look out into the Pacific Ocean. After dinner we walk on the Ventura beach, take off our shoes, and stroll through the sand, picking up seashells and admiring the beauty of this place.

After several weeks on the job, I am placed on the courts beat. I have a lot to learn, but back in Dayton I had covered some courts assignments and it doesn't take me long to get the hang of things. A newspaper war is being fought in the county. In Dayton, I was the only full-time police reporter in town. Here, I am one of a half dozen full-time courts reporters. The competition, both internal and external, is great and brings out the best in me. I write a lot of daily stories—nothing brilliant, but enough to fill our massive daily newshole. We have about a dozen *Times* reporters here in Ventura and six to eight pages to fill every day.

Despite the intensity of the job, I have more time to spend with Natalie and the kids than I had in Dayton. Since we are new to the area, we don't have the friends we have had in every other place we have lived. Natalie and I begin to immerse ourselves in our children's lives.

I start teaching Dwayne Jr., who is now seven, how to play basketball and baseball. We go to the park and shoot hoops, or out to the large patch of grass behind our townhouse and throw the baseball. He is somewhat skinny, like I was at his age. He learns these games quickly, but so does his sister, and she's only five. Christian hangs around us and won't let me show Dwayne how to play ball without giving her the same treatment. She puts on his baseball glove and attempts to catch the ball, but more often than not ends up getting hit with it. It's a hard ball, but she brushes off the injuries, even if they are to her face. She grits her teeth when she picks up a baseball bat and her determination is unbelievable.

C'mon, daddy, pitch me the ball, she says, her ponytail and colorful berets belying her actions. The ball comes, and she whacks it about seventy-five to one hundred feet. On the basketball court, as I'm showing Dwayne the art of the jump shot or how to dribble, this little girl is right there getting in between us.

Oooh, daddy, let me do it.

She shoots but has trouble getting the ball up to the rim.

Keep trying, honey, I say.

Dwayne Jr. joins a T-ball team coached by a Ventura narcotics officer. Coach Bob is patient with the kids and teaches them great fundamentals. The team goes undefeated, and Dwayne is one of the main players. We celebrate with Coach Bob and the other players and parents. The team is reflective of the melting pot that is Southern California; there are two black players, about a half dozen Latino boys, and six or seven whites. It dawns on me that we are all mostly middle class and have middle-class jobs.

I'm a reporter, Coach Bob is a cop, and one of my close friends, Pat, is a city prosecutor in Los Angeles. All my life, I have seen cops and prosecutors as the enemy, someone to fear. But now we all get along well because we have something in common: raising our kids in a safe neighborhood and giving them plenty of opportunities to reach their potential.

By early 1994, my kids start playing with two other black kids, a boy named Brandon, who is Dwayne Jr.'s age, and a girl named Fielding, who is six like Christian. These four little chocolate kids become inseparable. Christian and Fielding pull Fielding's wagon through our complex. Their wagon is filled with African-American dolls—and the two girls seem oblivious to the fact that they are apparently the only ones in the neighborhood with black dolls. They don't seem to care and neither do their blond, brunette, and red-haired friends.

Dwayne has just as much fun with Brandon as Christian does with Fielding. The two boys spend a lot of time at each other's house playing Nintendo. Brandon, beefy for his age, wears baggy pants and shirts and has a bright little smile. Dwayne is skinny and not yet into baggy-styled clothes. (Either that or his mother just refuses to buy them.)

Natalie and I never become great friends with Brandon and Fielding's parents, but we like them and they seem to like us. Brenda, their mother, brings over large bags of freshly picked fruit. Her husband, Dennis, and I stand outside late at night, under the lovely, starlit California sky, and discuss politics and sports. He thinks O. J. Simpson is innocent, like most of black

America. I think O. J. is guilty. Dennis at times marvels at my work.

I can't believe you're the same guy with his name in the paper every day, he says. By Dwayne Bray, he says, repeating my byline.

I just shrug.

Around here you wear shorts and a baseball cap and then I get the paper in the morning and there's your name. The same person.

I have a hard time figuring out his puzzlement. Anyway, I don't like to talk about work when I'm at home. But sooner or later we'll get into a conversation and he'll say, Did you read that story in the paper?

And I think, Not only did I read it, I wrote it.

It's a Saturday night, and Natalie and I are watching television when a news announcer interrupts the programming to tell us that a missing Ventura County nurse has been found dead. As courts reporter, I know that I will be handling the coverage of the murder trial if a suspect is caught. Within a week a nineteen-year-old man, Mark Scott Thornton, is arrested in Reno and charged with the nurse's murder.

Over the next eighteen months, I follow every detail of the case. Thornton is a troubled teenager who kidnapped the nurse, Kellie O'Sullivan, and took her to the Santa Monica Mountains, where he forced her into a grotto and shot her to death as she begged for her life. He stole her truck and proceeded to kidnap his ex-girlfriend in O'Sullivan's vehicle, a Ford Explorer.

At trial, Thornton's lawyers claim he has Attention Deficit Disorder and was abused as a child, but the jury finds him guilty of first-degree murder and sentences him to die. Before the judge rules on the sentence, I land the only one-on-one interview with Thornton, who, at twenty, will be Calfornia's youngest death row inmate in San Quentin if the judge doesn't overturn the jury's verdict.

I spend three hours in the Ventura County Jail talking to this young murderer through a glass partition. He admits he committed the crime but refuses to give details. He apologizes to the nurse's family for the pain he has caused.

We blow out the story and it runs in all editions of the *Times*. It is a coup for me, and my editors seem pleased.

Bill Overend, the city editor, calls me into his office and tells me that I will soon be getting duty in the *Times'* main office in downtown Los Angeles. He wants to know how I'm enjoying California life.

I think I will be here for a long, long time, I tell him.

◩

But by the spring of 1995, I am getting antsy. Natalie and I have made progress in pulling ourselves out of debt. We're not in the black, but at least we're moving in that direction. I start to think that I want bigger and better things that are hard to come by in California. I want a house, for instance, and property is too expensive here for me to afford anything decent. The most I could probably spend—if I could get a loan, that is—is probably one hundred thousand dollars. In California, that doesn't go very far.

I'm also feeling that it is going to take too long for me to get a shot at being a main player in the *Times'* downtown reporting operation. I like Ventura well enough; it's a great place to raise a family. With my impending temporary assignment in downtown Los Angeles, I have a shot at impressing the right people. But even if I make good on that opportunity, do I want to raise a family in Los Angeles County, a smog and crime haven where the traffic is relentless?

One of the most important drawbacks of living in California is that I am too far away to lend any real emotional support to my family in times of need. This first becomes apparent in October with the death of one of my grandma's older sisters, Aunt Willa. I want to be there for Grandma, but it is too expensive. Four months later, cancer gets the best of Uncle Son and he dies. I fly back to Ohio for the service. Unc had battled the disease for a while. It slowly ate away at his body and mind until he became almost senile. I hate the fact that I missed so much of the last year of his life. The whole experience repeats itself in June 1994 when my Uncle Bobby loses his fight with AIDS. My grandma has been there for me so often, but where am I all the times she needs me? After Bobby's death I feel I have let Grandma down by being so far away and not even attending the funeral.

Natalie, I say one day after work, I think I better start setting up some contacts back in the Midwest.

She agrees and my job search leads me back to Ohio. I have a chance to go home to Cleveland and write for the *Plain Dealer*. Or I can go to the *Akron Beacon Journal*. Or I can go back to Dayton, where I've been offered a job as an assistant metro editor. I choose Dayton because the pay is better and, if I am going into editing, it's better to do it in the city where I really cut my teeth as a reporter.

Moving back to Dayton not only puts me close enough to my family, it gives me the opportunity to start living out some of my dreams. I not only have a good job and a loving family, but as of October 1995, I have something else I've always wanted for my children: a house in the suburbs. Kettering is south of Dayton and a long way from East Cleveland. Its schools are among the finest in Ohio and that, along with affordable housing, is the reason we choose to live here. There are few other black families, and Natalie and I worry about making sure our kids don't lose their cultural identity. But that is probably a worry of families of all racial and ethnic persuasions. We believe strong families start in the household, and that's where Dwayne Jr. and Christian will learn their most important lessons.

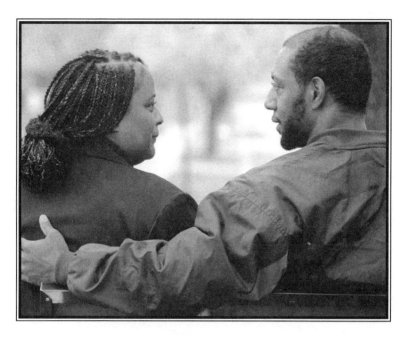

Natalie and I had many delicate discussions prior to the surgery.

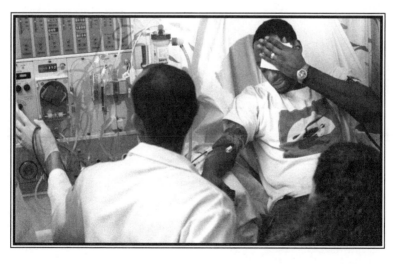

Charles, a dialysis tech, adjusts machinery as Calvin experiences cramping during treatment.

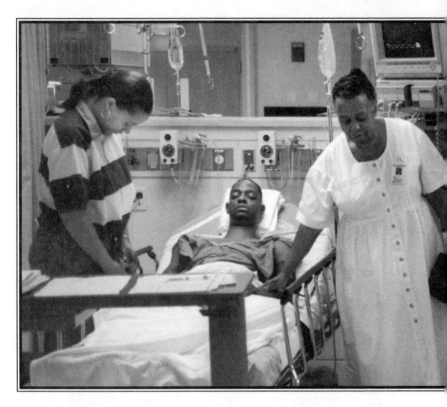

Before being taken to surgery, Calvin (left) and I are enveloped in prayer by his wife,

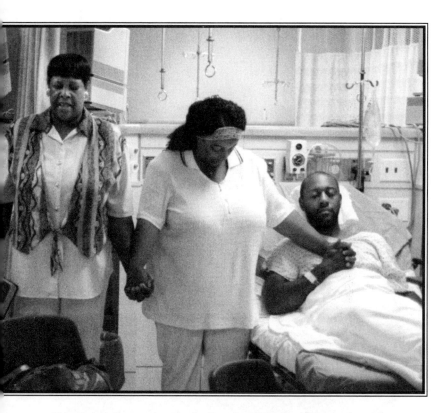

Misha (far left), his paternal grandmother, Emma Pearl Davis, Grandma Sangenella, and Natalie.

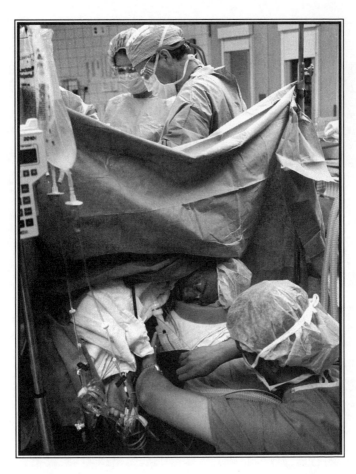

The anesthesiologist watches my face and monitors my vital signs during surgery.

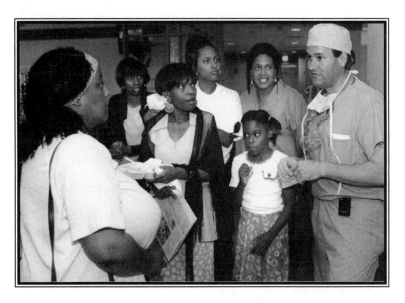

Dr. David Mulligan fills in the family after my kidney has been removed for transplant into Calvin.

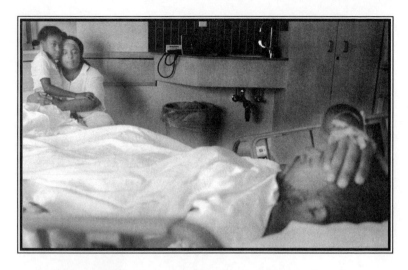

Christian and Natalie keep an eye on me as I start to feel the pain after surgery.

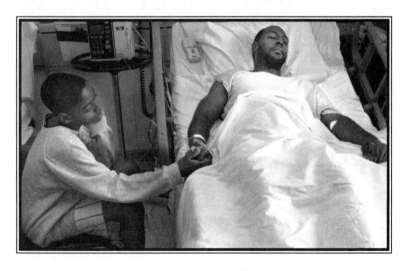

Dwayne Jr. tries to comfort me after surgery.

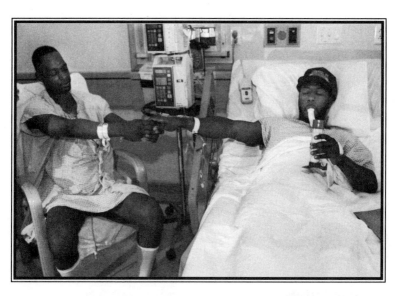

Calvin and I share a groggy moment two days after surgery.

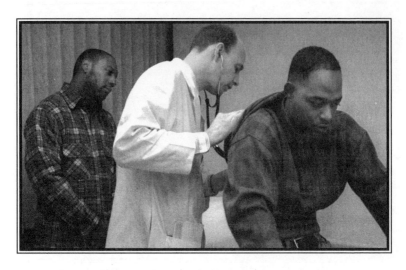

I keep a watchful eye as Calvin goes for his checkup three months after surgery.

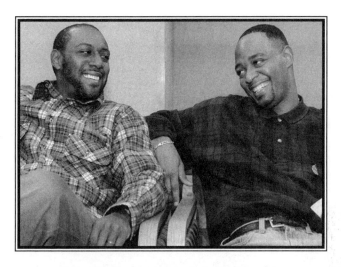

Calvin and I share a laugh three months after the surgery.

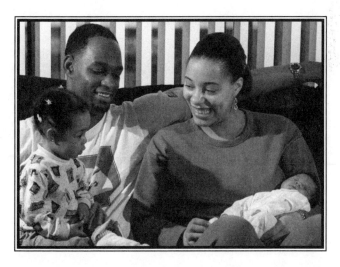

Calvin and his wife, Misha, enjoy a moment with their daughter Kalyn and infant son, James.

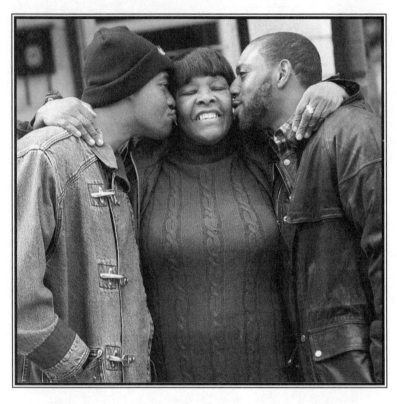

Calvin and I compete for Grandma's affections on Brightwood after surgery.

PART

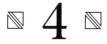

4

Tears stream down Little Calvin's face. Organ music blares from the speakers. Calvin is seated in the first row of pews at the Full Gospel Evangelistic Center on Martin Luther King Boulevard in southeast Cleveland. His father's body lies in a casket a few feet in front of him. It is July 5, 1996.

Natalie and I walk toward the front of the church, and I stop and embrace my first cousin. This is a terrible loss for Calvin. He is not only losing his father, but the one person in whom he could confide the most. From the time he moved in with his father back in the mid-1970s, Little Calvin has leaned heavily on Big Calvin to lead him through the landmines of growing up young and male at a time when the world around him is rapidly changing. Big Calvin was a hustler, but he also had a good grip on reality and knew what advice to give his son. Little Calvin had seen his dad get into trouble as well, and he learned from that, too.

Above all, Big Calvin was a loving man, someone we were lucky to know. The biggest weakness in the Brimage-Smith-Bray family has always been a strong male presence. Big Calvin, who had a baby with my mother's younger sister, was always different. When he was around, you felt like he was in charge of his destiny, whatever it might be; he controlled his own life. When things went bad for him, that was all right because he was only taking a risk, one that could pay off big time. When things went well, it was because he had planned and organized it that way. Big Calvin was the only man in our family who took time out for all the kids, whether he sired them or not. He would pull up in his Mercedes or Rolls Royce—cars he had acquired through whatever street hustle he had perfected—and load it up with us dirty, sweaty kids who had been out playing all day. Once he came by unannounced and took a bunch of us to the Geauga Lake Amusement Park in Aurora, Ohio. Another time, he came by and organized a softball game for anyone on Brightwood who wanted to play.

Come on, he said that day. Let's go play ball.

But Calvin, I said, We don't have but a few gloves and only one bat.

He laughed and said he would take care of that. We all drove to Silverman's department store, where he bought maybe a dozen new baseball gloves and a half dozen bats. At the counter, he pulled out a roll of bills topped off with hundreds.

Sir, said the cashier, I don't know if we can take those.

There's plenty more where they came from, Big Calvin told the woman. If you don't like those I'll just go to my banker and get you some more.

On the way to the park, the cops stopped Calvin, who was driving his gold Mercedes. I followed in one of his BMWs. They ran a check and found nothing, and we were on our merry way.

Later, Big Calvin said the patrolman did not know whom he had stopped.

If he would have taken me in and they knew what I've been up to, they would have made that cop a lieutenant, Calvin bragged.

Several months later, Big Calvin was behind bars. It was something as simple as not paying the bill on the BMW and refusing to return it. His money had run dry. He did six months for grand theft auto.

Of course, nothing illustrates his kindness more than his willingness to donate a kidney to his son in March 1991. The kidney never seemed to get going full strength, but for five years it worked well enough that Calvin continued a semblance of a normal life. In January 1996, however, the kidney died. Little Calvin was devastated, but he had known for a year now that the organ was losing steam. He was placed back on dialysis, and our family began to scramble for ways to bring back his health.

It's in the middle of this latest medical crisis that his father dies. As if he could take another blow, Little Calvin also has to deal with the fact that his mother, Pat, is on the lam from the law—and from a bounty hunter who frequently rings the bell on Brightwood looking for her because she has skipped bail as well.

A river of tears is pouring down Calvin's face as we sit here in the church, and I try to comfort him. I have not seen him this emotional before. Misha, his pregnant girlfriend and wife-to-be, is there to comfort him, too. So is Grandma.

After Big Calvin is buried and a few weeks pass, our family's attention shifts solely to Little Calvin and the dilemma of his health. He looks in bad shape—he's lost his skin tone and has dropped maybe forty pounds. Dialysis is no friend of his, just an acquaintance that helps him stay alive.

Calvin's options for a kidney transplant are failing one

by one. His mother is not a candidate for a transplant, even if she could be found: she has hepatitis and a nasty heroin habit. His father's sister has agreed to testing but is diagnosed with emphysema. His father's brother wants to help but is locked away in an Ohio prison and can't get approval for the operation from the Department of Corrections. Calvin has a half sister, Michelle, but the doctors warn her against considering donation because Calvin is still carrying their father's kidney. The mixture of Michelle's kidney and their father's could be volatile to Calvin's body.

So my first cousin, the closest person I have to a brother, is back where he started: no kidneys, and no donor available.

◫

As I follow each twist in Calvin's case, I rationalize. I manage to comfort myself with the thought that Calvin will receive a kidney from a cadaver—some good and kindly person who's made the proper mark on his or her driver's license, and whose untimely death might help a stranger live.

But then, as they always seem to, the facts get in the way of my contentment. I start researching the issue and come away glum. I find a plethora of books and articles on kidney disease and organ transplantation in the Dayton Public Library. I begin to spend a lot of my off-hours in the library, finding obscure research material in *Reader's Digest* and pulling information off the microfilm.

I find out that more than fifty-five thousand patients nationwide are awaiting transplants of all kinds, according to the list kept by the United Network for Organ Sharing. Every year, demand outstrips supply. Every year, the patient list grows.

To some degree, this shortage affects everyone—young and old, men and women, whites and blacks and Latinos, poor and rich, you and me, or someone we know. But it is more acute among certain segments of the population.

Around thirty-eight thousand of the patients on the list need kidneys. About a third of them, like Calvin, are black. Blacks are more than twice as likely to need kidneys because they are plagued with higher rates of diabetes and high blood pressure, the top two causes of kidney failure.

Blacks also wait twice as long to receive cadaver organs.

Black patients often receive organs from donors of other races and vice versa. But transplants aren't just about moving an organ from one body to another; they're about preventing the recipient from rejecting the strange organ. Although transplant patients take anti-rejection drugs for the rest of their lives, doctors still prefer to match organs within racial or ethnic groups to take advantage of tissue similarities, thereby further minimizing the risk of rejection.

◫

Can blacks donate at a higher rate? Of course. But cultural differences that may not occur to whites often get in the way of blacks donating. Many blacks mistrust the medical establishment, remembering such grievances as the Tuskegee, Alabama, experiments, where the U.S. Public Health Service withheld syphilis treatment for black men as late as the 1970s. They see wealthy white celebrities such as Mickey Mantle, David Crosby, and Larry Hagman get transplants quickly, and they figure their organs will go to the rich and famous. Some people are simply superstitious about surrendering part of their body.

What does all this mean to me?

I know that if Calvin were white, he might have to wait no more than a year for a cadaver kidney. As a black man, his wait is two to five years. I don't think he will last five years, let alone two; his blood has a tendency to clot easily, making the physical drain of dialysis even worse for him.

During my research, I find a statement that seems to sum up the controversy surrounding who gets organs and how quickly they get them. It is by Donald A. Streater, a representative to the United Network board of directors. He told a Congressional subcommittee: We can argue until hell freezes over about how to allocate organs, and that will not solve the problem. The bottom line is this— there are not enough organs.

Until now, I had known next to nothing about organ donation and the shortage of supply. Why should I? It had not affected me before. But suddenly it does.

Several months after Big Calvin's funeral, I drive from Cleveland for another major family event: Calvin and Misha are getting married. Now I'm thinking about the newlyweds and their infant daughter, Kaylin, and the unborn child Misha is carrying. What will the family's life be like without him? I know we can't wait several years to see if the government will move him up the waiting list so he can receive a kidney. I feel badly for him, but at the same time I have my own problems.

My cousin, like it or not, seems fated to be ground up in the bureaucratic gears of a national debate that shows no signs of resolution. And I am prepared to watch the system destroy him.

Then comes the call from Grandma.

Grandma calls with news I don't want to hear, just am not ready to hear.

Calvin was rushed into surgery during a dialysis treatment a few days earlier. The cause: a blood clot.

As I listen to Grandma's voice over the line, I begin feeling ill at the thought of doctors rushing to unhook the dialysis machines from my cousin, hurrying to stop the clotting and keep him from more serious danger.

My stomach turns. Guilt overtakes me.

I know my cousin needs a kidney, and now I feel as if I have abandoned him. I want someone else to help him. Maybe another family member. Maybe a government agency in charge of dispensing cadaver organs. But I have not stepped forward myself.

I know how long it will take for him to receive a cadaver kidney.

I know that dialysis can keep him going, but that living that way will be draining and difficult.

I know he could die.

I know, I know, I know.

Nothing else has worked for Calvin. I am thirty-two, relatively young, and healthy. God has given me two kidneys that function just fine. I have to give him one of mine.

He has never asked me to take such a step. Has never even hinted at it. But it is time, I know, for me to stop doing nothing more than just wishing the illness would disappear.

I decide all this during the conversation with my grandmother. Before she hangs up the phone, I tell her. She praises the Lord.

Natalie is at the grocery store. The kids are with friends. I try to figure out how to break the news to her of my weighty decision.

When her car pulls into the driveway, my heart starts racing. I hear the door shut and the sound of paper shopping bags brushing against one another.

I rush out a little too fast to help her with the groceries.

What's wrong? she says.

I hesitate as we make our way into the house and set down the bags.

I know you're not going to like this, but I have decided to see if I can donate a kidney to Calvin.

You're going to do what?! she screams. I don't blame her.

I just talked to Grandma. I explain what she said about the surgery and the emergency. About what lies ahead for him. Natalie argues that he has made it this far on dialysis.

He doesn't need dialysis! I say, my own voice rising. He's not going to make it long off dialysis. He needs a kidney! And I need to give him one of mine.

She is silent—forever, it seems.

But what about our kids, Dwayne? she says finally. Dwayne Jr. is ten; Christian is eight. If you give up a kidney, she asks, what happens if they need one down the road?

I hope they never need one, I mumble quickly, hoping to staunch the bleeding. And if they do, we'll cross that bridge when we get there.

Do whatever you want, Natalie says. I will support you because I'm your wife. I will be there for you. But don't expect me to agree with this decision.

◩

I know where Natalie is coming from. She has put up with a lot. Her family is different from mine; they are close but they don't necessarily believe in relying on each other as much. I come from a larger family that all counted on one another (my grandmother and seven of her brothers and sisters raised families in Cleveland), and now my aunts and uncles and cousins and I have kept up that same tradition. At times, the burden can fall on me disproportionately, for no other reason than that I am the only family member to have completed college. I have a white-collar job; most of my other close relatives are blue collar or unemployed. I have a stable nuclear family; most of them are in broken relationships with illegitimate kids. They are not married and don't have any real support systems. So it makes sense for them to count on me. I try to oblige, but Natalie, naturally, has a hard time comprehending my relationship with my relatives.

Her family operates differently. The basic reason is that she has only a small contingent of relatives in Cleveland. Both her father's and mother's families are dispersed throughout North Carolina, Alabama, and Michigan, as well as other places. So her family hasn't developed quite the same level of intense relationships that mine has.

◩

When the money calls come in from some of my relatives, Natalie turns the phone over to me. I more often than not give counsel, advice, or quick cash to the caller on the other end.

The calls come predominantly from Cleveland's East

Side, where Natalie and I grew up and where our families remain. But the calls also come from wherever Pat, Calvin's mother, might be: on the run from the law or in jail or prison; they come from my mother, who has been incarcerated in Texas prisons six times. They can come from almost anyone.

Natalie and I have made a better life for ourselves, but the money calls keep pulling us back. I don't mind. Natalie does. We have a different definition of what being a good family soldier is all about.

The money calls—a term coined by Natalie—come often enough to be a source of tension in my family life. We have made it out of the ghetto; we have worked and saved and are buying our own home in a middle-class suburb of Dayton. Our children are safe as they play in our quiet, tree-lined neighborhood, safe in one of Ohio's "top 100" school districts. I have a management job, and Natalie is able to stay home while our kids are young.

From the perspective of our extended family, we have a lot: a house, a car, good jobs, money in the bank, and a long-term marriage with two healthy children. Natalie is fully aware of how rich—how lucky—our little family looks to outsiders. She is fully aware and she is grateful. But she also knows how hard we have worked to get to this point. She wants to keep what is, by right, hers. She wants her family protected.

Natalie knows that I am different. We have been married for twelve years. We met as teenagers. I have tried never to turn my back on anyone who needs me, and I am needed a lot. Money is often borrowed, never to be seen again; the troubles of friends and relatives have often kept me awake at night.

But my biggest display of generosity comes without a request, without a phone call, before I hear any hint that

I might be needed. No one has asked me for this one. I have two working kidneys. Calvin has none. In my way of thinking, I'll just give him one of mine and everything will be fine. My cousin will have to accept this gift—he has to or he'll probably die, but he has never asked.

To Natalie, however, it is the same tired story. The old family is reaching out, clawing at the new family. They want, they need, thanks a lot, man, I'll pay you back. Always taking something.

This is my decision—Natalie knows that. Unbidden, unsolicited, I offer myself to my cousin. To Natalie, it is a direct threat to all she loves. Generous as she is in the community at our kids' school with her own time and talents, this still seems too much. What will happen to us if something happens to you? she asks.

It's the right thing to do, I believe. It's the only thing to do, I know. It's an important lesson for our children and Calvin's children, for everyone's children. If Dwayne Jr. ever needs a kidney, maybe Calvin's son will step forward. What goes around comes around.

There really is no choice, I tell her.

There's always a choice, Natalie thinks, and I have made mine. I know Natalie believes there is a lot of character behind my decision and that is the reason I have always made her proud.

She'll do what has to be done. But she knows that even with my ultimate offering, the money calls will never stop. Never.

◪

For months, I play a good game of phone tag with Penny Belden, the pretransplant coordinator at University Hospitals in Cleveland. She finally reaches me at the office in late July. Her voice is high-pitched and cheery.

She compliments me on my decision to be a donor, but she discourages me from getting my hopes up too high. The testing, she warns, will be precise and involved. The slightest problem could derail the process.

She showers me with information and questions.

What is my blood type? Penny asks. I don't even know. She sends me to my doctor to find out.

If Calvin and I have the same blood type, I will have to make the four-hour trip to Cleveland for a test matching our tissues. As Penny talks, I become dizzy with overload. She tells me about four or five other tests, including X-ray studies of my kidneys and more specialized blood and urine tests that will show if I am in good health and if my kidneys work well.

Medicare will cover the cost of the testing, she says, but it will not compensate me for time off work or for my trips to Cleveland.

These details, these logistics make my decision tangible. Suddenly, my willingness to donate a kidney is taking on physical meaning. A promise is becoming reality. I am making arrangements to allow strangers to cut into my body and take something from it.

I am afraid.

Like any sensible person, I've always had a healthy fear of needles. You will not find me in line at the office blood drive. If I want to donate a kidney, I will have to get over this. I will have to form intimate relationships with needles of all kinds.

My first such run-in comes on July 29, 1996, when I go to my doctor's office for the first blood test. I cringe as the nurse rolls up my sleeve and straps my left bicep. A vein emerges. She slides a needle into it. I watch blood shoot into the vial and tell myself all is well.

The sample goes to a lab in Cincinnati. Results will be sent to University Hospitals. I wait.

A week passes, then another. No word. Then a month. I want to phone Penny, but what if the news is bad? Maybe I am sick. My imagination wears itself out. I am a wreck.

One day in late October, Penny calls. My first question: What took so long?

That's not how it works, she says, setting me straight. You have to call me for results.

She tells me I have A-positive blood. So does Calvin.

I nearly leap from my seat. Don't get too excited, Penny cautions. This is just one hurdle, and there are plenty more. We schedule my tissue-typing test for December 9 at University Hospitals. Five weeks away.

I talk to Penny when I go up for the appointment, and she says something that surprises me: You should start thinking about a surgery date. We've still got a long way to go, but it's good to have a date ready.

N

Is there any history of high blood pressure in your family?

The question sounds simple. Marilyn Bartucci, head nurse and manager at University Hospitals' transplant center, is doing the asking. It is December 1996, my first trip to Cleveland for tests and the first time I meet the staff in the hospitals' transplant office.

Not that I know of, I say. I only know half of my family's history, medical or otherwise. I've never met my father.

I have to come to grips with a lot of personal and medical issues when I decide to be tested as a possible kidney donor. None, however, is tougher than questions about the paternal half of my family, the half I've never known.

For whatever reason, my father has never been in my life. I don't know why he wasn't—isn't—around. After a while, I don't care. My grandmother reared me in a house filled with love, my mother relating to me more as a big sister would.

But Bartucci isn't just prying; she has a good reason to ask about him. Hypertension and diabetes are silent killers that cause kidneys to deteriorate. If my father has a history of those diseases in his family, it would be an important factor in whether I can get by for the rest of my life on a single kidney.

I have decided that I will probably write about the experience of donating my kidney for the *Dayton Daily News* and have bounced the idea off my bosses at the newspaper. I am keeping notes and a journal, recording experiences, such as my meeting with Marilyn, that will be useful in telling the tale. But about this time, the kind of cosmic coincidence occurs that few writers or novelists would attempt, fearful of the reader's disbelief.

My father—suddenly and mysteriously after thirty-two years—tries to contact me.

Since I've been an adult, my mother and I have become distant. She has been a drug addict and moved to Houston, partly to be away from me, I suspect, so I won't see her in that condition. Now, however, she is out of prison and has been clean for three years. She is planning to be married and has a job as a telemarketer.

She knows about my decision to give a kidney to my cousin and comes to visit me in Dayton. We go to Cleveland for a few days to see family and friends, and, without my knowledge, she meets my father at a local restaurant. It is their first meeting since shortly after I was born.

Later that evening, my mother and I sit upstairs in my grandmother's house and she tells me she has seen him. His only purpose, she says, was to get me to call him—if I wanted to.

She hands me a torn piece of paper with seven digits on it: his phone number.

I do not want to call him, not now, not at this stage in my life. Where was he all those years? I don't want to seem bitter, but I am. It's not fair for a man to desert his children. There can never be an excuse for that.

Then I think about Marilyn and her questions about my family's medical history.

I can call this man, meet him, and at the very least, find out if there are any medical conditions in the family I should know about—especially before donating a kidney.

I place his phone number on the dresser mirror in my bedroom. Some mornings when I wake up, I stare at it. I want to know some things. A part of me even wants to see him. Curious, I guess. What does he look like? Is my thinning hair inherited? Is he smart? Athletic? What does he do for a living?

Hell, where has he been all my life?

I catch myself and just smile. I don't need to ask those questions. God has taken care of me all these years. He has been my true father.

I have the answers I need. Marilyn Bartucci will have to do without hers.

I don't remember what happens to the piece of paper. Maybe I tear it up, or just throw it away. Maybe it just falls off my mirror and onto the floor, and gets swept up with the rest of the trash.

◪

It doesn't take me long to figure out the pecking order at University Hospitals: from the bottom up, it's the technicians, then the nurses, and then most of the doctors. High above everyone else are the surgeons. The perception seems to be that they truly perform God's work, that they are more special.

By mid-March 1997, I have gone to Cleveland twice already to have blood work done. The results are encouraging—Calvin and I have similar genetics. Our blood is compatible. When it is mixed, the cells got along swimmingly, meaning less chance that his body will reject my kidney.

This is good news. As we move along in the process, I begin hearing more about the invisible surgeons: how they will handle our case, what they require of patients, how they have final say on the operation taking place.

But I wonder: If they are so darned important, why haven't I met them after seven months of testing?

I have met Penny Belden, the efficient pretransplant coordinator. I have met Marilyn Bartucci, the knowledgable nurse who manages the transplant center. I have met technicians who stick me with needles, take X-rays, and measure my vital signs. One even rubbed sticky jelly on my stomach for an ultrasound to determine the size and shape of my kidneys. And I have met Dr. Donald Hricik, Calvin's doctor. He says studies show that kidney donors, thirty years after the operation, live as normally as nondonors.

Like most others at the hospital, Dr. Hricik also speaks reverently of the surgeons. I think Mulligan will be doing your operation and Shulak will do Calvin's, he says during a March meeting with the two of us.

OK, so at least now I have names, which just makes me more curious. How long have they been at the hospital? What are their backgrounds? Hricik volunteers little more about them, but he does give me a preview of what surgery will be like. General anesthesia. An incision nearly from spine to navel, about eight to ten inches long. Slicing through muscle. The kidney is buried in the back under the rib cage, so that will be an obstacle.

The surgeon will have to cut off a small part of the rib. Or he might just spread the ribs apart and harvest the kidney that way.

Harvest. Harvest my kidney.

Hricik is directly before us, and Calvin and I sit so close in the small exam room that our legs brush together. The doctor is calm but frank. Transplant surgery, he says, is more traumatic for the donor than the recipient.

I want to faint. Earlier in the year, I injured my ribs playing pick-up basketball at the YMCA. The injury hurt like hell and took months to heal. I can't fathom someone cutting off a piece of one of my ribs—or, worse, using a tool to pry them apart.

I want to tell Calvin he has to find another donor. Or wait for a cadaver kidney. Then I look at Calvin. He is engaged in what Dr. Hricik is saying. Sitting on the edge of his chair. His hopes are high for the first time in years. He turns to me and shakes his head.

You hear that? he squeals. You still want to do this?

Before I can answer, Dr. Hricik orders Calvin to leave the room, so he can examine me.

I slowly disrobe. The doctor presses an icy stethoscope against my chest and back.

Breathe in . . . breathe out.

He presses his fingers against my genitals and orders me to cough. I am trembling. I feel like the teenager I once was, growing up in the inner city, anxiety a constant companion. My life—well ordered and sedate now, through the force of my own doing and that of my wife— seems to be spinning suddenly out of control.

Breathe in . . . breathe out . . . .
Breathe in.

◩

The grimace cuts across Calvin's face without warning.

He has been hooked to the dialysis machine for three hours, as usual, and everything seems fine. For about twenty-five minutes I have been there too, watching as he undergoes treatment. I have heard what dialysis is like, but now I am seeing it for myself.

The big, bulky machine pumps blood out of Calvin's body, filters it through a series of long, clear tubes, and cleans it. A huge, artificial kidney. I am amazed to watch blood flow through the plastic tubes, a crimson waterfall. Nature's work done the hard way.

Calvin is a veteran of these procedures. He even works as a technician in the hospital's dialysis unit. So he prefers to talk baseball. The Indians have made a big trade with the Braves this morning: Kenny Lofton for Marquis Grissom and David Justice. What are they thinking?

During the baseball banter, Calvin begins shifting uncomfortably in his chair. He frowns, I take a step or two back.

Charles! Calvin yells. My legs are cramping. Can you turn off the UF?

Charles Armstrong, a tall, thin technician in his early forties, rushes over and starts fidgeting with the machine. In no time, Calvin has cramps in his feet and toes.

I told him not to turn it on 64.5, Calvin snaps. I told him to put it on 66. I knew this was going to happen. I knew that this was too much. He didn't listen.

Since his last treatment Calvin has gained six pounds, all fluid. Normally, dialysis patients gain about three pounds between sessions, but Calvin missed his previous appointment because Misha just gave birth to their second child, and there have been problems. The baby, Calvin James, is jaundiced and has been kept in the hospital a few extra days.

Calvin's body does not care about his problems. The technician who has hooked him up to the machine, however, has tried to accommodate the situation. Wanting to rid Calvin of all the built-up fluid, he has set the dialysis machine too high, and it has been pulling too much fluid from his body at one time. Painful cramping can result.

And in this case, it does. Calvin was right.

Now Calvin is cramping all through his lower extremities—and a photographer from the newspaper and I are on hand to see it. The cameraman, Jim Witmer, is helping me document the transplant process. But his presence, and that of his clicking shutter, upsets the nurse who hustles to massage the cramps from Calvin's calves. She orders Jim to stop shooting.

Jim wants to capture both good and bad. Cramps have become part of the story, and he doesn't want the nurse interfering. It is Calvin's story, not hers.

Jim keeps his camera trained on Calvin and keeps clicking away. The nurse, kneeling and massaging, turns toward us.

DON'T TAKE ANOTHER PICTURE—AND I MEAN IT!

Jim doesn't move. He asks me, Should I keep shooting? What do you want me to do?

Here I am, a journalist and a donor, a writer and a patient, my paper's reporter and Calvin's cousin. Work and family have intertwined as never before. As Calvin writhes, the work on him continues—and yet it is plain that Jim's work and mine is, at that moment, a distraction. An obstacle to his care.

The cramp has moved and worsened. Calvin massages his left calf as Bonnie, the nurse, works his right leg so hard it looks as though it might come off.

As she works, she keeps her eyes on Jim.

I hesitate. I want to be able to show in our stories how dialysis is hard and how the patients who undergo it are brave. I want Jim to do his job as he sees fit.

Calvin and Bonnie knead Calvin's throbbing legs.

Jim, I say. We've got enough pictures.

In the afternoon, as he and Calvin and I have lunch, Jim is quietly frustrated. She was playing photo editor, he says. It's not up to her if I take pictures. It's up to you two. He points to Calvin and me. He never makes me feel bad about the decision. In truth, however, I feel that the further we go, the less any of what is happening is up to me.

◪

It is the time of trips and testing. A lot, too much, of both.

From December 1996 to May 1997, I travel half a dozen times to Cleveland for tests. Five hundred miles roundtrip each time.

Mostly the testing is routine stuff: blood, urine, X-rays. One test, called an arteriogram, is more involved and uncomfortable; the doctors run a catheter through an incision in my thigh, shoot dye at my kidneys, and X-ray them to see how well they work.

Everything has checked out fine for so long that it seems strange, almost funny, to have a poor result. But a blood test shows that I am secreting too much creatinine, a waste byproduct of the muscles. It is something my kidneys should take care of and it can signal trouble. Dr. Hricik orders me to undergo further testing and X-rays. Another trip.

Everyone is worried. Did I have kidney problems myself? I drive to Cleveland's University Hospitals, come back to Kettering, and anxiously await the results. Again.

Penny Belden, the pretransplant coordinator, calls with bad news, but not the bad news I expect: My paperwork has been marked incorrectly, she says, apologizing. I have been given the wrong test.

So I have to leave my wife and kids—again—to drive to Cleveland to get retested. More interstate, more mile markers.

And, happily, I receive different results. These show that each of my kidneys functions at 50 percent capacity, which means I have 100 percent kidney function and can be a donor. I am told that if one of my kidneys is removed, the other one will get used to doing all the work and kick in at 100 percent capacity.

After getting the word from Penny, I call Calvin to share the news that I have a clean bill of health. We are both excited. Now it is Calvin's turn to get a final physical before we can proceed.

Of course there are problems.

Calvin calls me on May 22. The doctors say I might have hepatitis C, he says. They can't go along with the transplant until they do a biopsy of my liver. They're trippin', talking about how it can be life threatening. He suspects it is a false reading, something having to do with the fact that he works in the dialysis unit, around blood all day.

The biopsy is put off several times and finally, on June 10, the results are back.

Calvin calls and says, The doctor says he saw a little inflammation but no fluid. I was nervous. What have I done to deserve liver problems? And the doctors are joking, Your liver is bad, Calvin. We can do both a liver and kidney transplant at the same time.

Kidding aside, we know we have dodged another bullet. Then on July 3, five days before our surgery is scheduled, the doctors find that Calvin is bleeding internally.

Calvin sounds worried over the phone, again. This news means one of three things: ulcers, colon cancer, or just constipation.

If it is either of the first two, the surgery will be called off, and he will face a new danger. Calvin is holding out for the best, but there is exasperation in his voice when he reaches me this night.

I definitely don't think I've got colon cancer and I definitely don't think I've got ulcers, he says over the phone. I just found out about this at 6 o'clock.

Strangely, the new round of tests to find the cause of the bleeding will parallel the final tests leading up to the still-possible transplant surgery. In our ongoing medical Never-Neverland, we will be taking our final tissue-matching tests in just four days, while awaiting the outcome of other tests.

One set of results, and I will head home to Dayton and back to my work-a-day world, knowing that I have given it my best.

Another set, and I will prepare to be knifed.

I have grown used to this game of medical high drama.

It has been almost a year since testing started. The transplant already has been postponed twice—once because the surgeons weren't available and again because of Calvin's liver biopsy. Through all the bumps in our road, pretransplant coordinator Penny Belden tries her best to keep my spirits up because she knows I'm getting frustrated with all the delays.

I'm excited, she chirps during one pep talk.

I am in a grousing mood. Why? I ask.

Because I like taking care of people.

Yeah, and she doesn't get sliced open doing it, either.

◩

On the Sunday before the transplant is scheduled, church seems like a very good idea. Calvin and I decide to go to Burning Bush Baptist Church with Grandma. We've been brought up in it, and everybody seems happy to see us. The people pray that Calvin will be able to get one of my kidneys.

Burning Bush is set in the heart of Cleveland's East Side in an old building painted fresh yellow and white. Grandma, who always gives more than she has, has donated fifteen hundred dollars to repave the parking lot. She helped start the church three decades ago and was on the committee to pick the only pastor it has ever had: Reverend Lee James Jones, who baptized me when I was about five, and who has presided over just about every important event in my family.

Today, no more than sixty parishioners show up on any given Sunday. There used to be more, including Calvin and me many years ago, but now the congregation is mostly gray and dwindling.

On this morning, Reverend Jones stands at the altar as the congregation's members come forth to pray for us, the transplant patients. Some people will give you some money, Jones preaches, wading through the kneeling people. Some people will give you some food. He takes a deep deliberate breath after every statement. But not everyone will give you one of their organs.

Amen! shouts Grandma.

Lawdy, Lawdy, Lawdy, look after 'em, says a short, gray-haired man in a rumpled suit.

These cousins love each other, Jones says in a drawl. I've known these boys since they were babies, and they have always been good boys, looking after their grandmother.

Now, as they embark on their latest journey, the Lord will be with 'em. Watching over 'em.

Preach it, Reverend! a woman who hasn't come up to the alter hollers, thrusting her arms skyward and falling excitedly into the grasp of an usher.

Calvin's eyes are clamped tight. His head rests on his bent knee. I look around and bow my head.

The Lord apparently hears our prayers. Later the next day, Penny reaches me around 6 P.M.—about thirteen hours before the set time for the surgery.

I just want to let you know everything is on for tomorrow, she says. The bleeding the doctors had to pinpoint in Calvin's body was caused by nothing more than constipation, a common minor ailment for dialysis patients who have to limit their fluid intake. All is well.

We are on.

Penny's happiness is infectious, even through the phone. She says, We passed a couple of great big hurdles today, Dwayne.

◪

The grandmothers join hands, bowing their heads.

The aunts and the wives join in, praying for their boys, their husbands.

Calvin and I are calm, half drugged, prepped, and prepared for our surgeries.

Lord have mercy. Calvin has been through this before with his father. When his father gave up a kidney, it was to save the life of his child. No parent would do less. No one has questioned that gift, not for a second.

Today he is here with me. This gift is harder to accept, open to question. Calvin hasn't been sure he should let me do it. But he does, because he has so little choice. It has taken nearly a year for the tests to be run, the details worked out. Here in Cleveland at University Hospitals, and now, Tuesday, July 8, 1997, it is about to happen.

Calvin is tired—he has been exhausted for months. Dialysis can only do so much, and keeping him alive was its only goal. Feeling good is an expendable option, never achieved. Calvin is alive, but far from well, far from healthy.

Within hours, though, he will have a real kidney, a one-owner, low-mileage organ that will cleanse the toxins from his body the way nature intended. If all goes well, he'll feel better immediately.

Calvin sits in his bed, eyes closed, holding the hand of Misha, now his wife of ten months.

Natalie stands by my bed, silently supportive, while Grandma calls on God to watch over her family. Emma Pearl Davis, Calvin's paternal grandmother and an ordained minister, reads from *Psalm 27*:

> *The Lord is my light and my salvation; whom*
> *shall I fear?*
> *The Lord is the strength of my life; of whom*
> *shall I be afraid?*

Monitors beep in the background; nurses go about their duties in the huge room reserved for those ready for surgery.

The group around Calvin and me is solemn, listening and believing as the Reverend Davis speaks about faith and love and Jesus Christ.

Amen. Amen. Natalie stands by me, her head bowed with the rest, but she is not part of this. She is separate; this is not her family. The extended support system belongs to Calvin and me. She is an outsider, married into this group of strong, outspoken women. She isn't blood, and therefore her voice, powerful though it is, is not always heard.

In a family of strong women, best interests aren't always the same. I am donating a kidney against Natalie's better judgment. She has come with me to Cleveland, of course, to support me, but she continues to question whether I've made the right choice. She is terrified.

Amen.

Natalie turns her head and wipes a tear. She turns back, squeezes my hand, and kisses me. There is no more she can do.

It is a routine operation, the doctors have assured everyone. Major surgery, but run-of-the-mill. Our transplant team has performed hundreds of such operations. No big deal.

Calvin and I are taken to our neighboring operating rooms, and the family heads to the hospital's waiting area for what they've been told will be several hours.

Dwayne Jr. and Christian are there. They are missing track practice, maybe even a meet, and this doesn't make them happy. They love running, and they are very, very good at it. They would probably rather be home in Kettering, secure in their summer routine.

But they never say so. One look at their mother and they know better than to complain. They are learning what you do for your family. They are being taught that you be there, and you stay, and you wait, because you're needed. Because it's your family.

Women come, women go, reading newspapers and

magazines, drinking pop, exchanging news and opinions. They are laughing and joking, teasing each other and reminiscing, while each one, in her own time, offers up silent pleas that all is going well.

◩

The anesthesiologists have it the toughest: They see the faces.

When the surgeons go to work, their subject's humanity—face, fingers, toes, anything identifiable as a person, anything with a name and a family—is draped off, out of sight, invisible. While they work, they see only the immediate area.

The anesthesiologists watch the monitors. And the faces.

Doctors Rajiv Tewari and Sheila Vaz gently cover my mouth with a mask, giving me no choice but to breathe their drug. Within seconds, I am out, unconscious, paralyzed. Many people fear surgery not because of the cutting, but because of the anesthesia, which takes a human being far too close to death. In seconds, I am at their mercy. I can't breathe.

Tewari and Vaz move with hurried precision, carefully and quickly inserting a tube into my mouth and down toward my lungs. It seems to take forever.

Don't worry, says a nurse, seeing the panic on an observer's face. If they don't get it in right away, they'll stop, give him some oxygen, and try again.

With the tube in place—on the first try—the doctors relax a bit and begin the job of monitoring the myriad flashing machines surrounding their work area, the area around my head.

The nurses strap me to the table, tucking rolled-up towels around my body to prop me up as I'm turned on my side, facing the wall, giving the surgeons better access to my kidney.

Dr. David Mulligan refers to X-rays before he cuts, judging the placement of the right kidney. Kidneys are well protected by the body, covered by several layers of muscle, located deep under the ribs; harvesting one is quite a chore. Mulligan bends down and begins work on the only part of me he can see, a circle of skin about a foot in diameter. He makes his incision, and an assisting resident follows the knife with a rag, mopping up the blood.

After the first cut, there is very little bleeding. Mulligan and his crew are trying out surgical scissors that cauterize as they cut, sealing the wound immediately as it forms. The scissors buzz and burn, cutting through my flesh as if it's filet. Each gauze rag is placed in a container. The post-surgical weight of the container will determine the amount of blood lost. In my case, it's hardly any. Mulligan is clearly in charge, but he's joined by Dr. James Merlino, a first-year resident, Dr. Melissa Reigle, a fourth-year resident, and Pat Abouhassan, a student from Wright State University's medical school in suburban Dayton. George Young is the circulating nurse, answering the phone and running the errands; Chuck Blinsky is the scrub tech, controlling the instruments. Everyone is relaxing, and everyone loves working with Mulligan. He's not just competent; he's affable, fair, and easygoing. For a surgeon.

There's music, which runs to classic rock. Mulligan doesn't pick these Eagles and Queen tunes—Young is just playing what this particular operating room has available, CDs others left behind.

Mulligan and crew slowly cut me nearly in half, slicing through three layers of muscle. They move carefully, layer by layer, until they can get at the kidney. It's a huge incision that will leave an eight-inch scar distinctive to kidney donors. It takes a good long while, then the doctors are deep inside, clamps holding the gaping wound open. They begin to cut my kidney away.

◻

Dr. James Shulak, Calvin's doctor, checks in periodically. How's he doing?

Great. Just fine. The doctors give Shulak, who's biding his time, an idea of when he can expect to go to work.

When the kidney is wrested free, it's put in a stainless steel bowl, covered with a towel and handed to Shulak, who walks it out the door and into his theater, right next door. He and resident Dr. Jeff Hazey sit at a table and flush my kidney over and over, cooling it down, washing it out, sealing off the unnecessary veins.

Calvin lies on his back, unknowingly awaiting the implant. There's only one place for this kidney to go; two original kidneys and a previously donated one have all failed, but they remain in his body. They do no good, but they do no harm; removal is an unnecessary intrusion. My right kidney will be inserted into the right side of Calvin's groin.

The doctors are happy with my donation—it looks terrific, they say—and talk about their previous transplant experiences.

They get excited anticipating the pinking when the kidney is hooked up to Calvin's circulation. When the organ goes to work—which is immediately, they say—there will be urine all over.

It's a beautiful sight, says Shulak.

About an hour into the operation, Shulak tenses. He yells for the newspaper photographer, who is in the room, to stop taking pictures—the mood in the room chills. There's a hole in the artery and repairing it will delay everything. It's not a disaster, but every minute counts. Shulak and Hazey work quietly, stitching the tear. When it's repaired, they relax a bit and continue sewing my connections into Calvin's body.

Then they're done. They wait for urine all over, but nothing happens. Shulak gives it a tap and waits. They're patient, but they're concerned.

The hole reparations are probably the cause of the delay in kidney function, but as the doctors stand idly by, it becomes clear all over again how fragile, how miraculous, how unbelievably bizarre this procedure is. The doctors wait, because they can't do anything else.

From here on out, it's up to Calvin's body and my kidney. They close Calvin's body and prepare to wait some more.

◻

Dr. David Mulligan—young, bright, and charismatic— arrives after removing my kidney. Word had spread that Mulligan was the doctor who'd taken care of Mickey Mantle's liver transplant—a celebrity surgeon has worked on me.

It looks good, Mulligan told the gathered family members. It went perfectly, he assures. The kidney has passed to the other half of the transplant team, headed by Dr. James Shulak, which will place it in Calvin's body, hook it up, and let nature take its course.

Two hours later, Dr. Shulak walks in. Calvin is fine, he says, but Shulak wants them to know about a problem. He had to repair a hole in the artery feeding the kidney, putting the surgery behind schedule and causing a few tense moments.

The kidney isn't up and running yet—they had hoped it would be—and it was possible the delay will result in some complications. It is equally possible that all will be fine. We'll just have to wait and see.

The family hangs on his words, then begins to speak: Where is the hole? How did it get there? Is he really OK? What does this mean? Behind their questions hangs the unspoken doubt: Are you telling us the truth?

◫

Dwayne couldn't have been living with a hole in his artery, Shulak says. It happened when the kidney was being removed or when it was being prepared, or when it was being placed in Calvin's body. He doesn't say it, but the implication is clear. One of the surgeons, or one of the surgeons' assistants, is responsible.

He is sure everything will be fine.

◫

Calvin and I are in recovery.

Calvin's kidney isn't working, and it is quite possible he'll need another round of dialysis until his new kidney kicks in. If his new kidney kicks in.

I am conscious, barely, and unbelievably groggy, unsure of who is in my room or what they are saying. My wife and children are there. Dwayne Jr. and Christian are unnaturally quiet, their eyes rarely leaving me. I am weak, bedridden, and I am slurring my words. They don't know this man. But they stay, and they stay quiet, and they watch.

I am not in pain yet, but I am assured a little too often that the pain will come and that it will be excruciating. It is early in the afternoon, and I need to sleep.

The next morning, the nurses report with pride that Calvin has made urine—and not just a little, eight quarts. That is good, they say. That is very, very good. Spirits rise as word spreads. Eight quarts! It's terrific.

Calvin and I are in private rooms across the hall from each other. Visitors wander in and out, our phones ring, Mike Tyson is on the television responding to the decision fining him for biting an opponent's ear. Calvin has been awaiting this news—he is a huge boxing fan and loves the spectacle of a Tyson fight.

Calvin's eyes are clear, his color bright. He feels a thousand times better, he says again and again. It is that simple and that complex: a kidney that works makes all the difference.

◩

The day after the surgery, my pain arrives with a vengeance. The nurse frowns, not with disapproval, but with concern. I am asking for more and more morphine, and the nurse says she'll page the pain team.

The two-man pain team arrives, identifiable by the "No Pain" badges on their white lab coats. They gently ask questions, nodding and making notes on their clipboard. They assure me that I am not imagining things; they stress (again) how very painful this operation is known to be. They assess my agony by asking for my rating: How bad is it from one to ten?

By noon, it is easily a fifteen. My dosage is maxed out. My body has adjusted.

Neither Calvin nor I are in any shape to travel, even by wheelchair, even across the hall, the day after surgery. The second day, rumors swirl that Calvin will be brought to my room for a visit.

Late that afternoon, Calvin and Misha shuffle across the hall, dragging IVs and catheters and medical paraphernalia with them. Calvin sits by my bed. We hold hands, mumble sentiments, act brave and embarrassed all at once.

Calvin takes a look at the huge basket of get-well gifts that have arrived for me today.

You got all that? he asks. All I got was a kidney.

I close my eyes and laugh. Oh, it hurts.

And it feels so good.

☒

What I need is a way to keep my mind off the pain. The first two days are hard. I have a catheter in my bladder, a device of almost unimaginable discomfort. On top of that, the swelling from my eight-inch incision is causing incredible itching in my back and thighs.

At one point, as I am trying to keep my mind off all that, I hear a nurse shout, Anesthesia! Anesthesia! Anesthesia!

I peer into the hallway and see white-suited medical personnel scrambling. They run into the room right across from mine. Calvin's room.

Get a doctor! someone yells. Someone closes my door. Panic seizes me: Calvin has to be rejecting the kidney. I ring the nurses, but they are too busy to respond.

Through the door, I can hear the commotion of nurses and doctors running in and out. Life-saving machines beeps every few seconds. The ruckus lasts fifteen minutes. Finally, a nurse cracks open my door.

What happened? I ask.

We had an emergency. We lost a patient.

I am silently stunned until she says, It wasn't your cousin.

It was another transplant patient, but I never get the details of the person's death. And it occurred just a few yards from where I lay healing.

N

Sometime later, a group of medical residents stop by. One begins undressing my wound. As he does, another strikes up a conversation.

Are you the writer?

Yeah, I say.

You know what you should write about? says the resident, a black man the others call J. J. The disparity in minorities giving kidneys.

His full name is John Jasper. He is from Cleveland Heights, where Calvin lived as teenager. I don't know what the numbers are, he says, fiddling with his stethoscope, but Dr. Mulligan tells me there is a disparity in that area.

I hate to say this, he continues, but with all the black-on-black violence, the murders, the killings, we could use some of those organs. They are very valuable. They can help save lives.

He lowers his head, as though ashamed to give voice to such a grisly truth.

I need to catch up with my group, J. J. says. He begins to walk away.

Hey, J. J., I say. He turns and looks at me. I'll try to get the word out, I promise.

N

Today I get to go home.

It's been five days, long and hurtful, in the hospital recovery ward. Now it's Saturday, July 12. Bright and warm. And today I get to go home.

Getting there, however, will not be easy. The main snag: two of the women closest to me are at each other's throats. Natalie thinks my grandmother is being too bossy when it comes to my care.

Grandma has suggested I stay in Cleveland at her home for at least a week after my release from the hospital. She wants Natalie to stay there with me. Natalie and I want to get back to Kettering, back to our own interrupted lives.

When Dr. Mulligan, my surgeon, assures me it is OK to make the drive home, Grandma is none too pleased. She has visited me in recovery a few nights before my scheduled release. The next night, after I tell her I'm not staying in Cleveland, she stays away. She approaches Natalie instead.

Your grandmother wants to know why I am taking you back to Dayton, Natalie says. I just told her, Mrs. Smith, he's my husband.

I know Grandma will not let a comment like that just ride. She loves me too much not to fight for what she thinks is right. She fought off the welfare caseworkers when they tried to farm me out for adoption thirty-two years earlier. She fought for me to go to school when I was on the threshold of teenage unruliness in a ghetto neighborhood. All her life, she has fought for my well-being. Now will be no different.

But Natalie has fought for me as well. Without her support, I know I would probably still be back in the old neighborhood—merely subsisting, like the vast majority of my childhood friends. She encouraged me to stick with college. She moved all over the country with me when I changed newspaper jobs. She is the mother of my two children.

I know I am lucky to have Natalie and Grandma,

especially at a painful time like this. But I can't stand that they are at odds, with me too weak to intervene. And how has Grandma responded to Natalie's defiance? She warns, If you take him home in his condition, you might not have a husband very long.

Perhaps she's overreacted. We'll be careful, and 225 miles in the car will not kill me.

But Lord, who knew about all these darn bumps in the road? Or that when you've got a fresh, eight-inch incision in your side, you feel each and every one?

We haven't been on Interstate 71 very long before I almost cannot bear it. Does Ohio have the most rippled, atrocious highways on the planet? I swear it does.

Don't hit that bump! I yell, as Natalie tries valiantly to dodge one pothole after another.

Finally I take a pain pill, recline the seat of the Explorer, and doze off. When we pull into our driveway, I crawl out of the car, into the house, and into bed. For the better part of a week, that's where I stay. When I am awake, it hurts so much that I scarf down a pill and slide back down into delicious, palpable, pain-free sleep.

Until I run out of pills.

The hospital has sent me home with only twenty painkillers. In a panic, I call Dr. Mulligan's office in Cleveland, but all they can do is mail me another prescription. I go three days on nothing more than Tylenol 3. These are not good days.

But then, too, they are. I am home, in my own house, my own bed. Eating my wife's good cooking. Watching *Jeopardy!* with my kids. Looking out the window at my dog. Nothing beats being home. And nothing beats the call I get from Calvin two days after arriving back.

I'm going home today, too, he says.

◩

Recovery is painful. But I'm afraid that I will become addicted to the painkillers, so after the first week post surgery I take only Tylenol 3. Four weeks after surgery, I return to work.

It's seems like I haven't been in the newspaper building for years. I walk with a slow gait past Carlos, the chief of security, who is manning the front entrance.

Dwayne, that was a nice thing you did, he says.

I wave, acknowledging his statement. I catch the elevator to the third floor of the newsroom, as I have hundreds of times before. I am foggy as I get off and enter the newsroom past the front clerk's station. People see me. They have heard about the surgery. Gary Weaver, a clerk in the sports department, slowly rises from his chair. I can see Gary even though he is about thirty feet away. There are many desks in between us but my eyes lock with Gary's. He stands, slowly, and starts to clap. Pretty soon others do the same.

I have never been this embarrassed. I have always liked energizing the newsroom with hot stories, but this isn't a story. This is real life. The incision in my side tells me so. It hurts at this moment. It stings.

Yet my colleagues are standing and applauding. All the managers hear this and they slowly walk out of their offices and they, too, applaud.

I have never been so embarrassed and yet so proud.

◩

It's four months after the surgery, November 1997, and Calvin is a different man—and not just because my kidney has given him back his health. The first transplant, his father's kidney that failed after five years, came to a younger, immature man who worried and wondered and couldn't sit still.

This time, he knows better. This time, he has faith.

The routine hasn't changed that much from the time of his first transplant: medication (a multicolor batch of pills morning, noon, and night to stave off organ rejection), regular blood tests, and doctor visits. The difference is determination to turn the big concerns over to God.

It's all in His hands anyway, Calvin says, when anyone asks him about his health.

It helps to have grandmas that reinforce the faith, he says, grandmas who are saved. They give him strength, a strength that's passed around.

It may help that Calvin is married now to Misha, whom he's known since high school. It may help that they have two children, eight-month-old Calvin Jr. (Little Man) and nearly two-year-old Kalyn, who, though too young to comprehend the seriousness of their dad's disease, know something was going on.

Calvin is different, too, at work. He takes care of things at the University Hospitals' dialysis center, where he spent so much time hooked up to machines himself. He says he can be a big help because he's been there, knows what's going on. He works at a place full of bad memories, but keeps good thoughts regardless. He says he doesn't let it bother him.

Grandma says she wishes he would take it a little more easy, but Calvin grabs hours when he can, working four twelve-hour shifts in a row, if he's needed.

And when he heads home, he always stops by Grandma's house, just to get him a kiss.

When he does that, Grandma tells him, Go on home! Get some rest yourself!

But Calvin stops by every night, even though sometimes Grandma is asleep. Calvin just goes into her bedroom and gets himself a big kiss.

Natalie is no longer worried about my short-term health. However, I think she will always be worried about my long-term prognosis.

She never wanted me to have this surgery, out of love and respect for me more than anything else. Her view will probably never change, until she sees me live for at least forty years after the surgery.

Frequently, when the kids are asleep and I'm lying in bed, she will take her finger and rub it across my scar.

Stop, I say, that tickles.

That's dead skin there, she says.

I wonder if it will always feel funny like that or if, with time, it will regain some feeling.

It will always be like that, she says.

These are little conversations, but at least she and I can talk about the surgery.

Our relationship is no different than it was before the surgery, before the biggest disagreement of our marriage, which is at fourteen years now. In the year following the transplant, we have continued to take family vacations, dote on our two children, and love one another.

In fact, I think our disagreement has made our love stronger because our marriage survived it.

I have a lot of respect for her. I think she is a terrific mother and a brave lady. I wrote about the surgery for the newspaper and a lot of our readers agreed with her position on the transplant. Wives say they would not want their own husbands to donate an organ to a loved one, especially someone who is not the donor's immediate relative such as a sister or brother or mother or father.

Not everybody agrees, however. Natalie says that she was in the store once and a woman came up to her and said, When I first started reading about your husband's story I thought you were the most selfish person I had ever seen.

I don't think Natalie is selfish. In fact, she's very giving. She gives her time to her family and her job, and allows me to give time as well. But she is also protective. Maternal instincts cause her to be that way. Above all, she wants to protect her family from harm's way. And for that, I cherish her.

◨

Grandma always says, God is good. Yes, He is.

It is ten months after the surgery. I am in Cleveland on Brightwood. Calvin comes over and says that he has just returned from a check-up. He says that all the vital measurements show his kidney working as well as someone who has never had—or needed—a transplant.

Give me hug, big cousin, he says.

I hug him but I want to really test his health.

You up for a game of hoops? I ask.

We drive over to our Aunt Marie's house. There is a basketball hoop up in the backyard. We choose teams. It's Calvin, our younger cousin Little Anthony, and me. We are playing three of our other relatives, including Andre, my younger cousin who was at the center of the scuffle Jerome and I had years earlier.

Andre is now six foot one and can jump out of the gym. He is definitely the best player on the court. I can't keep up with him. Calvin decides to guard him.

Are you sure? I say.

Yeah, c'mon, let's play ball, Calvin says.

I am more interested in seeing if he will be able to run and jump and keep up with Andre, who is nineteen and as healthy as a triple-crown winner. On the first play I throw the ball in to Calvin, who fakes left and drives to his right and scores. He looks over at me and winks.

I haven't seen him make moves like that on the basketball court since he was in high school. We go on to beat Andre's team by a bucket.

The final score is less important to me than the fact that I now know that as long as Calvin takes his pills on a regular basis, he will be able to lead a full and normal life. I am convinced of that now.

◪

Grandma is sitting on her bed talking to me. We are reminiscing about our family and how the welfare caseworker wanted her to put me up for adoption some thirty-three years ago. It is the day after Calvin and I played basketball. We are going through pictures, and she is telling me about our family tree, from her mother, Mattie Shields, to her brothers and sisters and her own marriages. We talk about her children and how they came into the world and eventually her grandchildren, of which I am the eldest.

That's when she thinks back to that day in November 1964, when she caught the bus downtown to see the caseworker. It was several weeks after my birth. Grandma has forgotten many things between then and now. But she remembers that day as clearly as if it were yesterday.

The woman kept saying, Mrs. Brimage, how you gonna

take care of this baby? Grandma remembers, tears welling up in her eyes. I told them the Lord was going to take care of us.

And He did.

EPILOGUE

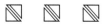

My wife and I were talking recently about our families and how they helped shape us. Natalie and I were born just a few hours apart at hospitals on Cleveland's East Side. She was born into a nuclear family structure, having a mother, Ola, a father, Nathaniel, and a brother, George.

Her parents eventually divorced, but even with the estrangement that brought to the family, the basic family unit was already in place: a mother, father, son, and daughter. Natalie's extended family was rather small. Her father is originally from North Carolina and had no siblings or parents in Cleveland. Her mother is from Alabama, and only her mother's father and three sisters were also in Cleveland.

My Cleveland family tree was much larger and more complex. My father was never in my life, and I grew up without sisters and brothers. But my maternal relatives more than filled the void. I was raised in the house on Brightwood with my mother and her seven brothers and sisters, as well as my grandmother, her husband, and her brother. They left me little time to be lonely. And then when my uncles and aunts began having children, there were frequently as many as a dozen or more of us living under one roof at any given time.

This meant that we counted on each other for all kinds of support. I also learned to substitute these relatives for the missing pieces of my own nuclear family. With my mother being so young, my grandmother became a mother figure. With my father absent, my grandmother's husband or my own maternal grandfather became my father figure. With no siblings, I was thrilled when a neighborhood friend would introduce me to others as the "brother" of one of my mother's siblings—instead of as their nephew.

In our house, we kids looked after each other and offered help whenever and wherever we could. If my mother needed someone to walk me to school because she was still in high school herself, her sisters Dorothy and Marie and Pat pitched in. When Dorothy, Marie, and Pat had children, Bill, Bobby, Antmo, and I offered to baby-sit. When Anthony grew older and sired kids of his own, it was the children of Dorothy and Marie who gave a helping hand.

Many people in America find this set-up strange and dysfunctional. Major institutions in this country still operate as if everybody grows up in a Cleaver-esque household—even though teen pregnancy is at an all-time high and the divorce rate is well over 50 percent. Banks still ask for my mother's maiden name when I access my accounts. My mother had the same last name before and after I was born. She didn't get married until I was thirty-two.

For many of the same reasons, I have always dreaded visits to the doctor. Invariably, a nurse asks about my father's health. For a time, I'd make up answers. I'd just substitute my grandfather in place of my missing father, figuring my grandfather and I had close enough genes.

So when I was asked if my father had diabetes, I'd say yes because I knew my grandfather was diabetic. When I was asked if my father had high-blood pressure, I'd say no because I didn't believe my grandfather had hypertension. This was a dangerous game, but one I just recently quit playing.

At times, I have wondered what it would have been like to grow up in a so-called normal family. To have had a father at my Little League games. To have had a mother in the Parent-Teacher Association. To have had a sister for whom I could chase the boys away.

Of course, I wouldn't trade my life and upbringing for any of that. When I think back to how I was raised and the positive influences of my grandmother then and my mother today, I know I have been blessed with a life that is as instructive as it is challenging and fun. I learned plenty that has allowed me to grow and prosper and appreciate raising my own children in the warmth of a nuclear setting.

I learned the responsibility one has to the broader family, and it is that sense of duty that motivated me to give Calvin the gift of a lifetime.